*a*ROMATHERAPY

A definitive guide to essential oils

L i s a   C h i d e l l

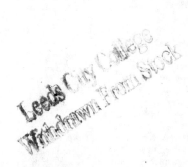

Headway • Hodder & Stoughton

Dedication

To my family and friends
my heaven-sent Rosie
my soul-sister Tara
and a special acknowledgement to Mr F. R. Brown.

British Library Cataloguing in Publication Data

Chidell, Lisa
  Aromatherapy; a definitive guide to essential oils
  1. Title
  615.8

  ISBN 0-340-56332-X

First published 1992
Impression number 10 9 8 7 6 5
Year   1998 1997 1996 1995

Typeset by Rowland Phototypesetting Limited, Bury St. Edmunds, Suffolk.
Printed in Great Britain for Hodder & Stoughton Educational, a
division of Hodder Headline Plc, 338 Euston Road, London NW1 3BH
by Athenæum Press Ltd, Gateshead, Tyne & Wear.

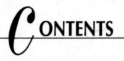ONTENTS

Introduction   1
Index of Essential Oils   5
Index of Conditions   69
Base Oils   95
Methods of Using Pure Essential Oils   99
Alphabetical Index of Conditions   105
Index of Essential Oils by Family and
   Principal Chemical Constituents   117
Useful Addresses   123

There is no incurable condition from which someone, somewhere, has not fully recovered

Lee J. Rose

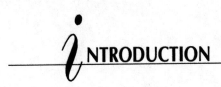

INTRODUCTION

This book is designed as a handbook to essential oils for the practitioner and interested lay person alike. It is intended as a supplement to existing literature and therefore contains no lengthy explanations or introductions, only the basic information required to assess which oils are beneficial in the treatment of a particular condition.

The book is divided into two main parts. The *Index of Essential Oils* includes information on the method of extraction, volatility*, principal chemical constituents and country of origin as well as a subjective description of the colour and aroma of each. The general and specific therapeutic properties of each oil are then listed exhaustively (the main uses being highlighted) and any contraindications are noted. (*Volatility has been described by the terms Top, Middle and Base note: a Top note oil being the most volatile with an aroma lasting for approximately 24 hours and being largely stimulant in effect; Base note oils being the least volatile, with an aroma which lasts up to one week and being largely sedative in effect.)

The *Index of Conditions* contains over 300 conditions which can be relieved or alleviated by essential oils. This section is divided into eleven subsections:

General properties of essential oils
Conditions related to the circulatory system
Conditions related to the digestive tract
Emotional conditions
Conditions related to the genito-urinary tract
Conditions related to the endocrine system
Conditions related to the head
Conditions related to the muscles and joints
Conditions related to the nervous system
Conditions related to the respiratory tract
Conditions related to the skin

Each condition has a list of recommended essential oils.

In addition there are notes on base oils and methods of using essential oils.

*i*NDEX OF ESSENTIAL OILS

Basil	7	Juniper (Berry)	38
Benzoin	8	Lavender	40
Bergamot	9	Lemon	42
Black Pepper	10	Lemongrass	43
Cajeput	12	Mandarin	45
Calendula (Marigold)	13	Marjoram (Sweet)	45
Camphor	13	Melissa	47
Caraway	14	Myrrh	48
Cardamom (Cardamon)	15	Myrtle	49
Cedarwood	16	Neroli	50
Chamomile (Camomile)	17	Niaouli	51
Cinnamon (Leaf)	19	Orange	52
Clary-sage	20	Patchouli	53
Clove (Bud)	21	Peppermint	54
Coriander	22	Petitgrain	55
Cypress	23	Pine (Needle)	56
Eucalyptus	25	Rose	58
Fennel (Sweet)	27	Rosemary	59
Frankincense	28	Rosewood	61
Garlic	30	Sage	62
Geranium	31	Sandalwood	63
Ginger	33	Tagetes (Marigold)	65
Grapefruit	34	Tea-tree (Ti-tree)	65
Hyssop	35	Thyme	66
Jasmine	37	Ylang-ylang	68

b

BASIL

Family:	Labiatae (Mint family)
Genus:	Ocymum basilicum
Country of origin:	Comoros
Extraction:	Distilled from leaves
Volatility:	Top note
Principal constituents:	Methyl chavicol (40–50 per cent) linaloöl, cineol, pinene and camphor
Colour:	Yellowish
Aroma:	Spicy, like aniseed
Contraindications:	Use in low concentrations as it may cause irritation Do not use during pregnancy.

GENERAL PROPERTIES:

Antispasmodic, stimulant, tonic, uplifting, warming

THERAPEUTIC PROPERTIES: (main uses underlined)

Circulatory:	Malaria
Digestive:	Colic, dysentry, flatulence, gastroenteritis, indigestion, intestinal infections, loss of appetite, nausea, stimulates digestion, vomiting
Emotional:	Anxiety, confusion, depression, exhaustion, fear, hysteria, indecision, insomnia, panic, paranoia, poor concentration or memory, run down, shock, stress
Genito-urinary:	Menstruation – absent, irregular or scanty periods
Glandular:	Stimulates adrenal cortex
Head:	Earache, fainting, headache, loss of sense

of smell, migraine, nasal polyps, rhinitis, sinusitis, vertigo

Muscular:	Antispasmodic, arthritis, cramp, gout
Neurological:	Epilepsy, nerve tonic, neuralgia, paralysis
Respiratory:	Asthma, bronchitis, catarrh, colds (chronic), emphysema, hiccough, whooping cough
Skin:	Congested, fevers, insect bites and stings, insect repellent, oily, snakebite, tonic, warts

BENZOIN

Family:	Styracaceae (Ebony family)
Genus:	Styrax benzoin (Friars balsam)
Country of origin:	Indochina
Extraction:	From bark of tree (resinoid)
Volatility:	Base note
Principal constituents:	Benzoic acid, vanillin, cinnamic acid
Colour:	Dark brown
Aroma:	Heavy and sweet, like vanilla
Contraindications:	Do not take internally.

GENERAL PROPERTIES:

Relaxing, sedative, warming

THERAPEUTIC PROPERTIES: (main uses underlined)

Circulatory:	Heart tonic, low body temperature, poor circulation
Digestive:	Colic
Emotional:	Anxiety, exhaustion, grief, hysteria, insomnia, jealousy, run down, stress
Genito-urinary:	Cystitis, diuretic, fluid retention, leucorrhoea, PMS
Head:	Laryngitis, sore throat

Muscular:	Arthritis, fibrositis, gout, rheumatism, rheumatoid arthritis
Respiratory:	Asthma, bronchitis, catarrh, colds, coughs (dry or painful), flu
Skin:	Blisters, chapped, chilblains, cracked, deodorant, dermatitis, dry, irritable, mature, wounds

BERGAMOT

Family:	Rutaceae (Citrus family)
Genus:	Citrus bergamia
Country of origin:	Italy
Extraction:	Expressed from peel of fruit
Volatility:	Top note
Principal constituents:	Linalyl acetate, limonene, linaloöl
Colour:	Greenish-yellow
Aroma:	Musty lemon
Contraindications:	Do not use in high concentrations on the skin or before exposure to sun as photosensitisation can occur.

GENERAL PROPERTIES:

Analgesic, anti-cancer, anti-inflammatory, antiseptic (powerful), antispasmodic, antiviral, cooling, relaxing, sedative, uplifting

THERAPEUTIC PROPERTIES: (main uses underlined)

Circulatory:	High body temperature, stimulates production of white blood cells
Digestive:	Colic, colitis, flatulence, gallstones, gastralgia, gastroenteritis, indigestion, loss of appetite, stimulates digestion, worms
Emotional:	Anorexia, anxiety, depression, hysteria, insomnia, panic, stress
Genito-urinary:	Cystitis, diuretic, gonorrhoea, leucorrhoea, PMS, sterility, urinary tract

	infections, uterine cancer, vaginal irritation
Glandular:	Breast cancer
Head:	Dandruff, glossitis, halitosis, seborrhoea of scalp, sore throat, stomatitis, tonsillitis
Muscular:	Aching, antispasmodic
Respiratory:	Bronchitis, catarrh, cough (dry or painful), diphtheria, tuberculosis
<u>*Skin:*</u>	Abscess, acne, carbuncles, chicken pox, deodorant, eczema (weeping), fevers, herpes, irritable, lice, measles, obesity, oily, psoriasis, scabies, shingles, sweating, ulcers, wounds

BLACK PEPPER

Family:	Piperaceae (Pepper family)
Genus:	Piper nigrum
Country of origin:	India
Extraction:	Distilled from dried berries
Volatility:	Middle note
Principal constituents:	Piperine
Colour:	Colourless to pale green – yellowing with age
Aroma:	A little like clove, warm and spicy
Contraindications:	Use in low concentrations as it may cause irritation. Do not use in conjunction with chemotherapy in the treatment of cancer.

GENERAL PROPERTIES:

Analgesic, antispasmodic, detoxifying, stimulant, tonic, warming

THERAPEUTIC PROPERTIES: (main uses underlined)

<u>*Circulatory:*</u>	Anaemia, angina, hypotension, low body

	temperature, lymphatic congestion, poor circulation, spleen tonic
Digestive:	Acid stomach, cholera, colic, colitis, constipation, diarrhoea, dysentry, flatulence, food poisoning, heartburn, indigestion, loss of appetite, nausea, stimulates digestion, stomach tonic, vomiting
Emotional:	Aphrodisiac
Genito-urinary:	Cystitis, diuretic, fluid retention, urinary tract infections
Head:	Fainting, headache, quinsy, toothache, vertigo
Muscular:	Aching, antispasmodic, fibrositis, lack of tone, rheumatism
Respiratory:	Catarrh, colds, coughs, flu
Skin:	Cellulite, chilblains, fevers

C

CAJEPUT (Cajuput)

Family:	Myrtaceae (Shrubs and trees)
Genus:	Malaleuca leucodendron
Country of origin:	Indonesia
Extraction:	Distilled from leaves and buds
Volatility:	Top note
Principal constituents:	Cineol (45–65 per cent), terpineol, pinene and various aldehydes
Colour:	Greenish-yellow
Aroma:	Camphoraceous
Contraindications:	Use in low concentrations as it may cause irritation. **Niaouli** is a non-irritant alternative with similar properties.

GENERAL PROPERTIES:

Analgesic, antiseptic (powerful), antispasmodic, antiviral, fungicidal, stimulant, warming

THERAPEUTIC PROPERTIES: (main uses underlined)

Circulatory:	Poor circulation, stimulates immune system
Digestive:	Colitis, dysentry, gastritis, gastroenteritis, indigestion, vomiting, worms
Genito-urinary:	Cystitis, painful periods, urinary tract infections
Head:	Earache, laryngitis, sore throat, toothache
Muscular:	Aching, antispasmodic, arthritis, fibrositis, gout, rheumatism, rheumatoid arthritis
<u>*Respiratory:*</u>	Asthma, bronchitis (chronic), colds, pneumonia, tuberculosis
Skin:	Acne, insect bites and stings, wounds

CALENDULA (Marigold)

Family:	Compositae (Daisy family)
Genus:	Calendula officinalis
Country of origin:	Egypt
Extraction:	Maceration of petals
Colour:	Pale yellow
Aroma:	Negligible

GENERAL PROPERTIES:

Anti-inflammatory, fungicidal

THERAPEUTIC PROPERTIES: (main uses underlined)

Circulatory:	Varicose veins
Digestive:	Haemorrhoids, gastritis, gastroenteritis, indigestion, liver tonic, ulcers
Emotional:	Anxiety, tension
Genito-urinary:	Menopause, menstruation – irregular or painful periods
Muscular:	Arthritis, fibrositis, gout, rheumatism, sprains
Skin:	Acne, athlete's foot, bruises, burns, chapped, chilblains, cracked, dermatitis, eczema, inflamed, regenerative, ringworm, scars, stretch marks, thread veins, ulcers, wounds

CAMPHOR

Family:	Lauraceae (Laurel family)
Genus:	Cinnamomum camphora
Country of origin:	China
Extraction:	Distilled from a substance found in the wood of the tree
Volatility:	Middle note
Principal constituents:	Camphor, linaloöl, terpineol, pinene,

limonene, cineole, safrole, methyl
eugenol, caryophyllene, terpenes

Colour:	Yellowish
Aroma:	Mild eucalyptus
Contraindications:	A relatively toxic oil which should be reserved for use in acute conditions only. Do not use during pregnancy.

GENERAL PROPERTIES:

Analgesic, antispasmodic, balancing, sedative, stimulant, warming

THERAPEUTIC PROPERTIES: (main uses underlined)

Circulatory:	Heart tonic, hypotension, low body temperature, poor circulation, vasoconstrictor
Digestive:	Cholera, colic, constipation, diarrhoea, flatulence, gall stones, gastroenteritis, stimulates digestion, vomiting, worms
Emotional:	Anxiety, depression, hysteria, insomnia, irritability, panic, run down, shock, stress
Genito-urinary:	Diuretic, fluid retention
Head:	Toothache
Muscular:	Aching, antispasmodic, arthritis, fibrositis, gout, rheumatism, rheumatoid arthritis, sprains
Respiratory:	Asthma, bronchitis, colds, coughs, flu, pneumonia, tuberculosis
Skin:	Acne, bruises, burns, chilblains, fevers, inflamed, lice, oily, ulcers, wounds

CARAWAY

Family:	Umbelliferae (Parsley family)
Genus:	Carum carvi

Country of origin:	Holland
Extraction:	Distilled from seeds and crushed fruit
Volatility:	Top note
Principal constituents:	Carvone (50–60 per cent), limonene
Colour:	Yellowish
Aroma:	Warm and spicy
Contraindications:	Use in low concentrations as it may cause irritation. Do not use during pregnancy.

GENERAL PROPERTIES:

Antispasmodic, stimulant, warming

THERAPEUTIC PROPERTIES: (main uses underlined)

Circulatory:	Low body temperature, poor circulation, swollen lymph nodes
<u>*Digestive:*</u>	Abdominal distension, air swallowing, colic, flatulence, gastritis, indigestion, loss of appetite, nausea, stimulates digestion, stomach tonic, worms
Emotional:	Irritability
Genito-urinary:	Diuretic, fluid retention, menstruation – painful
Glandular:	Increases flow of breast milk
Head:	Dizziness, vertigo
Muscular:	Aching, antispasmodic, arthritis, gout, rheumatism, rheumatoid arthritis
Respiratory:	Pleurisy
Skin:	Scabies

CARDAMOM (Cardamon)

Family:	Zingiberaceae (Ginger family)
Genus:	Elettaria cardamomum
Country of origin:	India
Extraction:	Distilled from seeds

Volatility:	Middle note
Principal constituents:	Terpineol, cineol, limonene
Colour:	Colourless to yellow
Aroma:	Warm, spicy and sweet
Contraindications:	Use in low concentrations as it may cause irritation.

GENERAL PROPERTIES:

Antispasmodic, stimulant, tonic, uplifting, warming

THERAPEUTIC PROPERTIES: (main uses underlined)

Circulatory:	Low body temperature, poor circulation
Digestive:	Colic, flatulence, heartburn, indigestion, loss of appetite, nausea, stimulates digestion, stomach tonic, vomiting
Emotional:	Aphrodisiac, exhaustion, poor concentration, run down
Genito-urinary:	Diuretic, fluid retention, menstruation – painful
Head:	Halitosis, headache
Muscular:	Antispasmodic
Neurological:	Sciatica
Respiratory:	Bronchitis, catarrh, cough

CEDARWOOD

Family:	Pinaceae (Conifer family)
Genus:	Cedrus atlantica (Atlas)
	Note: Another variety of cedarwood is available – Juniperus virginiana. It comes from a different family of conifers (cupressaceae) but has very similar therapeutic properties to cedrus atlantica.
Country of origin:	Morocco
Extraction:	Distilled from wood
Volatility:	Base note

Principal constituents:	Cedrene, cedrol, cedrenol
Colour:	Colourless to pale yellow
Aroma:	Musty and woody
Contraindications:	Use in low concentrations as it may cause irritation.
	Do not use during pregnancy.
	Do not use in conjunction with chemotherapy in the treatment of cancer.

GENERAL PROPERTIES:

Anti-cancer, balancing, detoxifying, sedative

THERAPEUTIC PROPERTIES: (main uses underlined)

Circulatory:	Blood purifier, lymphatic congestion
Emotional:	Anxiety, hysteria, insomnia, panic, shock, stress
Genito-urinary:	Cystitis, diuretic, fluid retention, gonorrhoea, inflamed kidneys, kidney tonic, leucorrhoea, PMS, thrush, urinary tract infections
Head:	Alopecia, dandruff, laryngitis, seborrhoea of scalp, sore throat
Muscular:	Arthritis, gout
Respiratory:	Bronchitis, catarrh, colds, coughs, flu
Skin:	Acne, astringent, dermatitis, eczema, insect repellent, irritable, oily, psoriasis

CHAMOMILE (Camomile)

Family:	Compositae (Daisy family)
Genus:	Anthemis nobilis (Roman)
	Note: Other varieties of chamomile are available – ormenis mixta (Moroccan) and matricaria chamomilla (German, or blue chamomile). Both possess similar therapeutic properties to the Roman variety. German chamomile, however,

has a high azulene content making it
particularly effective in treating severe
skin conditions.

Country of origin:	France
Extraction:	Distilled from flowers
Volatility:	Middle note
Principal constituents:	Esters (85 per cent) and chamazulene
Colour:	Blue, turning green with age
Aroma:	Heavy, musty, apple-like
Contraindications:	Do not use in early pregnancy if a serious risk of miscarriage exists.

GENERAL PROPERTIES:

Analgesic, anti-allergic, anti-cancer, anti-inflammatory,
antispasmodic, relaxing, sedative, tonic, uplifting

THERAPEUTIC PROPERTIES: (main uses underlined)

Circulatory:	Anaemia, palpitations, spleen tonic, stimulates production of white blood cells, vasoconstrictor
Digestive:	Abdominal distension, colic, colitis, constipation, diarrhoea, dysentry, flatulence, gallstones, gastralgia, gastritis, gastroenteritis, indigestion, jaundice, liver congestion, liver tonic, loss of appetite, stimulates digestion, stomach tonic, ulcers, vomiting, worms
Emotional:	Anger, anxiety, depression, fear, hypersensitivity, hysteria, insomnia, irritability, jealousy, panic, shock, stress
Genito-urinary:	Cystitis, diuretic, fluid retention, haemorrhage, inflamed kidneys, kidney stones, kidney tonic, menopause, menstruation – absent, heavy, painful or irregular periods, PMS, urinary tract infections, vaginal irritation, vaginitis
Head:	Conjunctivitis, dandruff, dizziness, earache, fainting, gingivitis, headache,

migraine, mouth ulcers, mumps, oral
thrush, teething, tooth abscess,
toothache, vertigo

Muscular:
Aching, antispasmodic, arthritis, cramp,
fibrositis, gout, lumbago, rheumatism,
rheumatoid arthritis, sprains

Neurological:
Convulsions, nerve tonic, neuralgia,
sciatica

Respiratory:
Catarrh, coughs (tickly), flu

Skin:
Abscess, acne, allergies, animal bites,
boils, broken capillaries, burns, chapped,
chicken pox, cracked, dermatitis, dry,
eczema, fevers, herpes, inflamed,
irritable, measles, psoriasis, scars, sores,
stretchmarks, sunburn, supersensitive,
thread veins, tonic, wounds

CINNAMON (Leaf)

Family:	Lauraceae (Laurel family)
Genus:	Cinnamomum zeylanicum
Country of origin:	Sri Lanka (Ceylon)
Extraction:	Distilled from leaves
Volatility:	Base note
Principal constituents:	Cinnamic aldehyde, eugenol
Colour:	Pale yellow
Aroma:	Hot and spicy
Contraindications:	Do not use during pregnancy. Use only under the guidance of a professional aromatherapist. Do not use in conjunction with chemotherapy in the treatment of cancer.

GENERAL PROPERTIES:

Antiseptic (powerful), antispasmodic, detoxifying, haemostatic,
stimulant, tonic, warming

THERAPEUTIC PROPERTIES: (main uses underlined)

Circulatory:	Haemorrhage, hypotension, low body temperature, poor circulation
Digestive:	Abdominal distension, acid stomach, cholera, colic, constipation, diarrhoea, flatulence, gastralgia, indigestion, loss of appetite, stimulates digestion, worms
Emotional:	Depression, exhaustion, poor concentration or memory, run down
Genito-urinary:	Impotence, intramenstrual bleeding, leucorrhoea, sterility
Head:	Fainting, sinusitis, toothache
Muscular:	Antispasmodic, fibrositis, rheumatism
Respiratory:	Colds, coughs, flu, haemoptysis
Skin:	Astringent, bruises, insect bites and stings, lice, scabies, snake bite, tonic

CLARY-SAGE

Family:	Labiatae (Mint family)
Genus:	Salvia sclarea
Country of origin:	France
Extraction:	Distilled from flowers
Volatility:	Top note
Principal constituents:	Linaloöl, linalyl acetate
Colour:	Colourless
Aroma:	Sweet, floral and nutty
Contraindications:	Do not use during first six months of pregnancy. Do not use if alcohol has been consumed.

GENERAL PROPERTIES:

Anti-inflammatory, antispasmodic (powerful), antiviral, relaxing, sedative, tonic, uplifting, warming

THERAPEUTIC PROPERTIES: (main uses underlined)

Circulatory:	Hypertension
Digestive:	Colic, flatulence, indigestion, stimulates digestion, stomach tonic
Emotional:	Anxiety, aphrodisiac, depression, exhaustion, fear, hysteria, insomnia, irritability, panic, paranoia, run down, stress
Genito-urinary:	Diuretic, fluid retention, frigidity, impotence, kidney tonic, leucorrhoea, menopause, menstruation – absent, irregular or painful periods, PMS, sterility, thrush, uterine tonic
Head:	Conjunctivitis, sore throat, vertigo
Muscular:	Antispasmodic
Neurological:	Convulsions, nerve tonic, neuralgia
Respiratory:	Asthma, cough (convulsions), whooping cough
Skin:	Astringent, boils, deodorant, inflamed, insect bites and stings, mature, sweating, ulcers

CLOVE (Bud)

Family:	Myrtaceae (Shrubs and trees)
Genus:	Eugenia caryophyllata
Country of origin:	Madagascar
Extraction:	Distilled from flower buds
Volatility:	Base note
Principal constituents:	Eugenol (70–90 per cent), eugenol acetate, caryophyllene
Colour:	Colourless to pale yellow
Aroma:	Spicy and sweet
Contraindications:	Use only under the guidance of a professional aromatherapist.

GENERAL PROPERTIES:

Analgesic, anti-cancer, antiseptic (powerful), antispasmodic, antiviral, stimulant, tonic, warming

THERAPEUTIC PROPERTIES: (main uses underlined)

Circulatory:	Poor circulation, swollen lymph nodes
Digestive:	Abdominal distension, acid stomach, diarrhoea, flatulence, indigestion, nausea, stomach tonic, worms
Emotional:	Exhaustion, poor concentration or memory, run down
Genito-urinary:	Impotence, menstruation – absent or painful periods, sterility
Head:	Earache, sinusitis, toothache, vertigo, weak gums
Muscular:	Aching, antispasmodic, arthritis, fibrositis, gout, rheumatism, rheumatoid arthritis
Neurological:	Neuralgia
Respiratory:	Asthma, bronchitis, colds, flu, pleurisy
Skin:	Bruises, lice, measles, scabies, snakebite, sores, sweating, ulcers, wounds

CORIANDER

Family:	Umbelliferae (Parsley family)
Genus:	Coriandrum sativum
Country of origin:	Russia
Extraction:	Distilled from seeds
Volatility:	Top note
Principal constituents:	Coriandrol (d-linaloöl) – (60–65 per cent), pinene, terpinene, cymene, borneol, geraneol
Colour:	Colourless to pale yellow
Aroma:	Fresh, spicy and slightly sweet

Contraindications: Use in low concentrations as it may cause irritation.

GENERAL PROPERTIES:

Analgesic, antispasmodic, stimulant, warming

THERAPEUTIC PROPERTIES: (main uses underlined)

Circulatory:	Poor circulation
Digestive:	Abdominal distension, air swallowing, colic, colitis, flatulence, gastralgia, indigestion, loss of appetite, stimulates digestion, stomach tonic
Emotional:	Anorexia, depression, exhaustion, poor concentration or memory, run down
Muscular:	Aching, antispasmodic, arthritis, fibrositis, gout, rheumatism, rheumatoid arthritis
Neurological:	Neuralgia

CYPRESS

Family:	Cupressaceae (Conifer family)
Genus:	Cupressus sempervirens
Country of origin:	France
Extraction:	Distilled from leaves and cones
Volatility:	Middle note
Principal constituents:	Cedrol, d-pinene, d-camphene, terpinyl esters, cymene, terpenic alcohol
Colour:	Colourless to yellow
Aroma:	Woody and musty
Contraindications:	Do not use during the first four months of pregnancy. Do not use with hypertensives.

GENERAL PROPERTIES:

Anti-cancer, antispasmodic, astringent (powerful), cooling,

detoxifying, haemostatic, relaxing, sedative, tonic, uplifting, (anything with excess fluid)

THERAPEUTIC PROPERTIES: (main uses underlined)

Circulatory:	Blood purifier, haemorrhage, high body temperature, poor circulation, varicose veins, vasoconstrictor
Digestive:	Diarrhoea, dysentry, flatulence, haemorrhoids, liver congestion, liver tonic
Emotional:	Anxiety, bed wetting, confusion, grief, insomnia, irritability, stress
Genito-urinary:	Diuretic, fluid retention, haemorrhage, incontinence, intramenstrual bleeding, menopause, menstruation – heavy or painful periods, ovarian tonic, PMS
Glandular:	Balances female sex hormones, stops flow of breast milk
Head:	Gingivitis, laryngitis, loss of voice, mouth ulcers, nose bleed
Muscular:	Antispasmodic, arthritis, cramp, fibrositis, gout, loss of tone, rheumatism, rheumatoid arthritis
Respiratory:	Asthma, coughs (convulsive), emphysema, flu, haemoptysis, hayfever, whooping cough
Skin:	Astringent, broken capillaries, cellulite, chilblains, deodorant, dermatitis, eczema, fevers, insect repellent, mature, oily, sweating, thread veins, tonic

e

EUCALYPTUS

Family:	Myrtaceae (Shrubs and trees)
Genus:	Eucalyptus globulus
Country of origin:	Portugal
Extraction:	Distilled from leaves
Volatility:	Top note
Principal constituents:	Cineol (eucalyptol) (70–80 per cent), pinene, aldehydes, terpenes, globulol
Colour:	Pale yellow
Aroma:	Strong and camphoraceous
Contraindications:	Do not use in conjunction with chemotherapy in the treatment of cancer.

GENERAL PROPERTIES:

Analgesic, anti-cancer, antiseptic (powerful), antispasmodic, antiviral, cooling, detoxifying, haemostatic, stimulant, uplifting

THERAPEUTIC PROPERTIES: (main uses underlined)

Circulatory:	Blood purifier, haemorrhage, high blood sugar, high body temperature, malaria, palpitations, poor circulation
Digestive:	Cholera, diarrhoea, dysentry, gall stones, indigestion, typhoid, worms
Emotional:	Confusion, depression, exhaustion, run down
Genito-urinary:	Cystitis, diuretic, fluid retention, gonorrhoea, haemorrhage, inflamed kidneys, kidney tonic, leucorrhoea, menstruation – heavy or painful periods, urinary tract infections, uterine cancer
Glandular:	Diabetes

Head:	Headache, laryngitis, migraine, rhinitis, sinusitis, sore throat
Muscular:	Aching, antispasmodic, fibrositis, rheumatism, rheumatoid arthritis, sprains
Neurological:	Nerve stimulant, neuralgia
Respiratory:	Asthma, bronchitis (chronic), catarrh, colds, coughs (convulsive, dry or painful), diphtheria, emphysema, flu, hayfever, pneumonia, tuberculosis
Skin:	Acne, boils, burns, carbuncles, chicken pox, deodorant, fevers, herpes, insect repellent, lice, measles, scarlet fever, shingles, ulcers, wounds

f

FENNEL (Sweet)

Family:	Umbelliferae (Parsley family)
Genus:	Foeniculum vulgare
Country of origin:	Italy
Extraction:	Distilled from seeds
Volatility:	Middle note
Principal constituents:	Anethole (50–70 per cent), d-phellandrene, d-limonene
Colour:	Colourless to yellowish
Aroma:	Like liquorice
Contraindications:	Use in low concentrations as it may cause irritation. Do not use with epileptics, children under six or during the first five months of pregnancy. Do not use in conjunction with chemotherapy in the treatment of cancer. Use with care in treating breast or female reproductive system cancers.

GENERAL PROPERTIES:

Antispasmodic, detoxifying, tonic, warming

THERAPEUTIC PROPERTIES: (main uses underlined)

Circulatory:	Alcohol poisoning, blood purifier, lymphatic congestion, spleen tonic
Digestive:	Abdominal distension, colic, colitis, constipation, flatulence, food poisoning, gastralgia, indigestion, loss of appetite, nausea, stimulates digestion, stomach tonic, vomiting, worms
Genito-urinary:	Cystitis, diuretic, fluid retention, kidney stones, kidney tonic, menopause,

menstruation – absent, irregular or painful periods, PMS, urinary tract infections

Glandular: Increases flow of breast milk, similar effects to oestrogen

Head: Dizziness, gingivitis, weak eyesight

Muscular: Antispasmodic, arthritis, gout

Respiratory: Bronchitis, catarrh, flu, hiccoughs, whooping cough

Skin: Animal bites, bruises, cellulite, congested, insect bites and stings, obesity, oily, snakebite

FRANKINCENSE

Family: Burseraceae (Resinous trees and shrubs)
Genus: Boswellia carterii
Boswellia thurifera
Country of origin: North East Africa
Extraction: Distilled from gum of tree (resinoid)
Volatility: Base note
Principal constituents: Pinene, dipentene, p-cymene, camphene, d-borneol, verbenone, verbenol
Colour: Colourless to pale yellow
Aroma: Woody, spicy and slightly camphoraceous
Contraindications: Do not take internally.

GENERAL PROPERTIES:

Haemostatic, relaxing, sedative, tonic, uplifting, warming

THERAPEUTIC PROPERTIES: (main uses underlined)

Circulatory: Haemorrhage

Digestive: Colic, haemorrhoids, indigestion, stimulates digestion

Emotional: Anxiety, confusion, depression, fear, hysteria, indecision, insomnia, irritability, panic, paranoia, stress

Genito-urinary:	Cystitis, diuretic, fluid retention, gonorrhoea, haemorrhage, inflamed kidneys, intramenstrual bleeding, leucorrhoea, menstruation – heavy, PMS, uterine tonic
Head:	Laryngitis, nose bleed
Neurological:	Nerve tonic
Respiratory:	Asthma, bronchitis, catarrh, coughs, flu, shortness of breath
Skin:	Astringent, carbuncles, inflamed, mature, oily, regenerative, scars, stretchmarks, tonic, ulcers, wounds

g

GARLIC

Family:	Liliaceae (Lily family)
Genus:	Allium sativum
Country of origin:	Mediterranean
Extraction:	Distilled from bulb
Volatility:	Top note
Principal constituents:	Allicin, disulphides
Colour:	Yellowish
Aroma:	Very pungent (recommended as a dietary supplement in the form of oral 'perles')
Contraindications:	Do not use with irritable skin conditions or irritable digestive conditions, nor with dry or severe coughs.
	Do not take while breast feeding as may cause colic in the baby.
	Do not use in conjunction with chemotherapy in the treatment of cancer.

GENERAL PROPERTIES:

Anti-cancer, antiseptic (powerful), antispasmodic, antiviral, detoxifying, fungicidal

THERAPEUTIC PROPERTIES: (main uses underlined)

Circulatory:	Anaemia, arteriosclerosis, heart tonic, high blood cholesterol, hypertension, inflamed lymph nodes, malaria, palpitations, poor circulation, stimulates immune system, varicose veins
Digestive:	Abdominal distension, colic, colitis, diarrhoea, dysentry, gallstones, gastralgia, gastroenteritis, haemorrhoids, indigestion, intestinal infections, stimulates digestion, typhoid, ulcers, worms

Emotional:	Run down
Genito-urinary:	Cystitis, kidney stones, thrush, urinary tract infections
Glandular:	Balances thyroid secretions, goitre
Head:	Deafness, earache, sinusitis, tonsillitis, toothache
Muscular:	Antispasmodic, arthritis, cramp, fibrositis, gout, rheumatism, rheumatoid arthritis
Respiratory:	Asthma, bronchitis (chronic), catarrh, colds, diphtheria, emphysema, flu, hayfever
Skin:	Abscess, acne, athlete's foot, boils, chilblains, corns, fevers, insect bites and stings, obesity, regenerative, ringworm, scabies, ulcers, verrucae, warts, wounds

GERANIUM

Family:	Geraniaceae (Geranium family)
Genus:	Pelargonium graveolens
	Note: Other varieties of geranium are available – pelargonium odorantissimum and pelargonium capitatum (rose geranium). Both possess similar therapeutic properties to pelargonium graveolens, rose geranium having, as the name implies, a rose-like aroma.
Country of origin:	Morocco
Extraction:	Distilled from leaves
Volatility:	Middle note
Principal constituents:	Geraniol, citronellol, linaloöl, terpineol
Colour:	Pale green
Aroma:	Heavy, sweet, floral

GENERAL PROPERTIES:

Analgesic, anti-cancer, anti-inflammatory, balancing, haemostatic, relaxing, stimulant, tonic, uplifting, warming

THERAPEUTIC PROPERTIES: (main uses underlined)

Circulatory:	Haemorrhage, lymphatic congestion, poor circulation
Digestive:	Diarrhoea, gallstones, gastralgia, gastroenteritis, haemorrhoids, jaundice, liver tonic, ulcers
Emotional:	Anxiety, confusion, depression, exhaustion, hypersensitivity, hysteria, panic, poor concentration or memory, run down, shock, stress
Genito-urinary:	Diuretic, fluid retention, frigidity, haemorrhage, impotence, inflamed kidneys, intramenstrual bleeding, kidney stones, kidney tonic, leucorrhoea, menopause, menstruation – heavy, PMS, sterility, thrush, urinary tract infections, uterine cancer
Glandular:	Balances hormones, diabetes, mastitis, stimulates adrenal cortex
Head:	Conjunctivitis, dandruff, glossitis, laryngitis, mouth ulcers, oral thrush, stomatitis, sore throat, tonsillitis
Muscular:	Aching, lumbago
Neurological:	Neuralgia
Respiratory:	Colds, flu, haemoptysis
Skin:	Acne, astringent, burns, cellulite, chapped, congested, cracked, dermatitis, dry, eczema (dry), herpes, inflamed, insect repellent, lice, measles, oily, scars, shingles, stretchmarks, supersensitive, tonic, ulcers, wounds

GINGER

Family:	Zingiberaceae (Ginger family)
Genus:	Zingiber officinalis
Country of origin:	India
Extraction:	Distilled from root
Volatility:	Base note
Principal constituents:	Zingiberine, zingiberol, camphene, phellandrene, cineole, borneol, linaloöl, citral
Colour:	Pale green/yellow oil
Aroma:	Warm, spicy and sweet
Contraindications:	Use in low concentrations as it may cause irritation.

GENERAL PROPERTIES:

Stimulant, tonic, warming

THERAPEUTIC PROPERTIES: (main uses underlined)

Circulatory:	Low body temperature, poor circulation
<u>*Digestive:*</u>	Abdominal distension, colic, constipation, diarrhoea, indigestion, flatulence, loss of appetite, nausea, stimulates digestion, travel sickness
Emotional:	Depression, run down
Genito-urinary:	Painful periods
Head:	Quinsy, sore throat
<u>*Muscular:*</u>	Aching, arthritis, fibrositis, gout, rheumatism, rheumatoid arthritis
Respiratory:	Bronchitis (chronic), catarrh, colds
Skin:	Bruises

GRAPEFRUIT

Family:	Rutaceae (Citrus family)
Genus:	Citrus paradisi
Country of origin:	United States of America
Extraction:	Expressed from peel of fruit
Volatility:	Top note
Principal constituents:	Limonene, citral
Colour:	Pale yellow
Aroma:	Warm, fresh and fruity
Contraindications:	May photosensitise the skin if used before exposure to the sun.

GENERAL PROPERTIES:

Uplifting, tonic

THERAPEUTIC PROPERTIES: (main uses underlined)

Circulatory:	Blood purifier
Digestive:	Constipation, digestive stimulant, gall stones, liver tonic, stomach tonic
Emotional:	Depression, run down
Genito-urinary:	Diuretic, fluid retention, kidney tonic
Skin:	Cellulite, obesity

h

HYSSOP

Family:	Labiatae (Mint family)
Genus:	Hyssopus offincinalis
Country of origin:	France
Extraction:	Distilled from leaves and flowers
Volatility:	Middle note
Principal constituents:	Pinocamphone, pinene
Colour:	Yellowish
Aroma:	Spicy and fresh
Contraindications:	Use only under the guidance of a professional aromatherapist. Do not use during pregnancy. Do not use with epileptics or hypertensives.

GENERAL PROPERTIES:

Anti-cancer, antispasmodic, antiviral, relaxing, stimulant, tonic

THERAPEUTIC PROPERTIES: (main uses underlined)

Circulatory:	Heart tonic, hypotension
Digestive:	Abdominal distension, colic, colitis, constipation, flatulence, gall stones, gastralgia, gastroenteritis, indigestion, loss of appetite, stimulates digestion, worms
Emotional:	Grief, poor concentration or memory, run down
Genito-urinary:	Diuretic, fluid retention, inflamed uterus, kidney tonic, leucorrhoea, menstruation – absent or scanty periods
Head:	Earache, quinsy, sore throat
Muscular:	Antispasmodic, fibrositis, rheumatism, rheumatoid arthritis, sprains

Neurological:	Nerve tonic, neuralgia
Respiratory:	Asthma, bronchitis (chronic), catarrh, emphysema, shortness of breath, tuberculosis, whooping cough
Skin:	Astringent, bruises, dermatitis, eczema, fevers, wounds

j

JASMINE

Family:	Oleaceae (Olive family)
Genus:	Jasminum grandiflorum
	Note: Another variety of jasmine, jasminum officinale, is available which possesses very similar therapeutic properties to jasminum grandiflorum.
Country of origin:	Morocco
Extraction:	An absolute extracted from flowers by enfleurage
Volatility:	Base note
Principal constituents:	Benzyl acetate (65 per cent), linaloöl, linalyl acetate, benzyl alcohol, jasmone, indole, methyl anthranilate
Colour:	Yellow/brown
Aroma:	Sweet, musky
Contraindications:	Do not take internally. Do not take in first four months of pregnancy.

GENERAL PROPERTIES:

Antispasmodic, relaxing, sedative, tonic, uplifting, warming

THERAPEUTIC PROPERTIES: (main uses underlined)

Emotional:	Anorexia, anxiety, aphrodisiac, depression, fear, hypersensitivity, hysteria, insomnia, panic, paranoia, run down, stress
Genito-urinary:	Frigidity, gonorrhoea, impotence, menopause, menstruation – painful, sterility, uterine tonic
Glandular:	Increases flow of breast milk, prostatitis

Head:	Laryngitis
Muscular:	Antispasmodic
Respiratory:	Asthma, catarrh, coughs, emphysema
Skin:	Allergies, dermatitis, dry, irritable, regenerative, supersensitive

JUNIPER (Berry)

Family:	Cupressaceae (Conifer family)
Genus:	Juniperus communis
Country of origin:	Yugoslavia
Extraction:	Distilled from berries
Volatility:	Middle note
Principal constituents:	Terpineol, alpha-pinene, cadinene, camphene, junene, camphor of juniper
Colour:	Colourless to green/yellow
Aroma:	Light, pungent
Contraindications:	Do not use in first six months of pregnancy. Use in low concentrations when treating severe kidney disorders. Do not use in conjunction with chemotherapy in the treatment of cancer.

GENERAL PROPERTIES:

Analgesic, antiseptic (powerful), antispasmodic, antiviral, balancing, detoxifying, relaxing, sedative, stimulant, tonic, uplifting, warming

THERAPEUTIC PROPERTIES: (main uses underlined)

Circulatory:	Arteriosclerosis, blood purifier, haemorrhage, high blood cholesterol, hypertension, low body temperature, lymphatic congestion, poor circulation, spleen tonic, varicose veins

Digestive:	Cholera, colic, colitis, diarrhoea, dysentry, flatulence, haemorrhoids, indigestion, liver cirrhosis, loss of appetite, stimulates digestion, stomach tonic, typhoid
Emotional:	Anxiety, aphrodisiac, fear, hysteria, insomnia, panic, paranoia, run down, stress
Genito-urinary:	Cystitis, diuretic, fluid retention, haemorrhage, inflamed kidneys, inflamed uterus, intramenstrual bleeding, kidney stones, kidney tonic, leucorrhoea, menstruation – absent, heavy, painful or scanty periods, PMS, sterility, urinary tract infections
Glandular:	Diabetes
Head:	Dandruff, seborrhoea of scalp, toothache
Muscular:	Aching, antispasmodic, arthritis, fibrositis, gout, lack of tone, rheumatism, rheumatoid arthritis
Neurological:	Epilepsy, nerve tonic, paralysis
Respiratory:	Catarrh, colds, coughs, flu, haemoptysis
Skin:	Acne, astringent, boils, carbuncles, cellulite, deodorant, dermatitis, eczema (dry or weeping), fevers, lice, measles, obesity, oily, psoriasis, regenerative, scars, snakebite, stretchmarks, thread veins, tonic, ulcers, wounds

l

LAVENDER

Family:	Labiatae (Mint family)
Genus:	Lavandula officinalis
	Note: Lavendin (lavandula fragrans) is a weaker alternative to lavender, particularly useful if a less sedative oil is required.
Country of origin:	France
Extraction:	Distilled from flowers
Volatility:	Middle note
Principal constituents:	Linalyl acetate, linaloöl, geraniol, lavandulol, pinene, cineol, caryophyllene, coumarin
Colour:	Colourless
Aroma:	Light and floral
Contraindications:	Do not use in early pregnancy if a serious risk of miscarriage exists. Do not use in conjunction with chemotherapy in the treatment of cancer.

GENERAL PROPERTIES:

Analgesic, anti-cancer, anti-inflammatory, antiseptic (powerful), antispasmodic, antiviral, balancing, cooling, detoxifying, fungicidal, relaxing, sedative, tonic, uplifting

THERAPEUTIC PROPERTIES: (main uses underlined)

Circulatory:	Anaemia, heart tonic, high body temperature, hypertension, lymphatic congestion, palpitations, poor circulation, spleen tonic, stimulates immune system, swollen lymph nodes, varicose veins
Digestive:	Abdominal distension, colic, colitis, diarrhoea, flatulence, gall stones,

gastralgia, gastroenteritis, indigestion, loss of appetite, nausea, travel sickness, typhoid, ulcers, vomiting, worms

Emotional:
Anxiety, depression, exhaustion, hysteria, insomnia, irritability, panic, poor concentration or memory, run down, shock, stress

Genito-urinary:
Cystitis, diuretic, fluid retention, gonorrhoea, inflamed uterus, kidney tonic, leucorrhoea, menopause, menstruation – absent, irregular, painful or scanty periods, PMS, thrush

Head:
Alopecia, conjunctivitis, dandruff, dizziness, earache, fainting, halitosis, headache, inflamed eyelids, laryngitis, loss of voice, migraine, mouth ulcers, nosebleed, oral thrush, rhinitis, sinusitis, sore throat, teething, tonsillitis, weak gums

Muscular:
Aching, antispasmodic, arthritis, fibrositis, gout, lack of tone, rheumatism, rheumatoid arthritis, sprains

Neurological:
Convulsions, epilepsy, nerve tonic, neuralgia, paralysis, sciatica

Respiratory:
Asthma, bronchitis (chronic), catarrh, colds, coughs (convulsive, dry, painful or tickly), diphtheria, flu, hayfever, pneumonia, tuberculosis, whooping cough

Skin:
Abscess, acne, allergies, animal bites, athlete's foot, blisters, boils, broken capillaries, bruises, bunions, burns, carbuncles, cellulite, chapped, chicken pox, chilblains, cracked, deodorant, dermatitis, eczema (dry), fevers, herpes, inflamed, insect bites and stings, insect repellent, irritable, lice, mature, psoriasis,

regenerative, ringworm, scabies, scars,
sensitive, snakebite, sores, stretchmarks,
sunburn, tonic, ulcers, wounds

LEMON

Family:	Rutaceae (Citrus family)
Genus:	Citrus limon
Country of origin:	Italy
Extraction:	Expressed from peel of fruit
Volatility:	Top note
Principal constituents:	Terpenes (95 per cent), limonene, camphene, pinene, geraniol, citral, linaloöl
Colour:	Pale green/yellow
Aroma:	Sweet and fresh
Contraindications:	Use in low concentrations as it may cause irritation or photosensitisation. Do not use in conjunction with chemotherapy in the treatment of cancer.

GENERAL PROPERTIES:

Acidity regulator, antiseptic (powerful), antiviral, detoxifying,
fungicidal, haemostatic, stimulant, tonic, uplifting

THERAPEUTIC PROPERTIES: (main uses underlined)

<u>*Circulatory:*</u>	Anaemia, arteriosclerosis, blood purifier, haemorrhage, heart tonic, malaria, poor circulation, regulates blood pressure, stimulates production of white blood cells, varicose veins
<u>*Digestive:*</u>	Acid stomach, air swallowing, colic, constipation, diarrhoea, dysentry, flatulence, gall stones, gastritis, heartburn, indigestion, jaundice, liver congestion, liver tonic, loss of appetite, typhoid, ulcers, vomiting

Emotional:	Depression, exhaustion, run down
Genito-urinary:	Diuretic, gonorrhoea, haemorrhage, kidney stones, kidney tonic, menopause, menstruation – heavy or painful periods, thrush
Glandular:	Diabetes
Head:	Conjunctivitis, dandruff, earache, glossitis, headache, laryngitis, migraine, mouth ulcers, mumps, nosebleed, oral thrush, quinsy, sinusitis, stomatitis, sore throat, tonsillitis, toothache, weak gums
Muscular:	Aching, arthritis, fibrositis, gout, rheumatism, rheumatoid arthritis
Respiratory:	Asthma, bronchitis (chronic), catarrh, colds, coughs, flu, hayfever, pleurisy, pneumonia, tuberculosis
Skin:	Acne, athlete's foot, blisters, boils, broken capillaries, cellulite, chapped, chilblains, congested, corns, fevers, herpes, insect bites and stings, insect repellent, lice, obesity, oily, regenerative, ringworm, scabies, shingles, snakebite, sores, thread veins, verrucae, warts, wounds

LEMONGRASS

Family:	Gramineae (Aromatic grasses)
Genus:	Cymbopogon citratus
Country of origin:	India
Extraction:	Distilled from grasses
Volatility:	Top note
Principal constituents:	Citral (70–80 per cent), myrcene (15–20 per cent)
Colour:	Yellow to red/brown

Aroma:	Strong and musty
Contraindications:	Use only under the guidance of a professional aromatherapist.

GENERAL PROPERTIES:

Antiseptic (powerful), stimulant, tonic, uplifting

THERAPEUTIC PROPERTIES: (main uses underlined)

Circulatory:	Poor circulation
Digestive:	Colitis, gastroenteritis, indigestion, stimulates digestion
Emotional:	Anxiety, hysteria, panic
Glandular:	Stimulates breast milk production
Head:	Headache, migraine
Muscular:	Lack of tone
Skin:	Acne, deodorant, fevers, insect repellent, oily, sweating, tonic

$\mathcal{M}$

MANDARIN

Family:	Rutaceae (Citrus family)
Genus:	Citrus reticulata
Country of origin:	Italy
Extraction:	Expressed from the peel of fruit
Volatility:	Top note
Principal constituents:	Limonene, methyl anthranilic acid, methyl ester
Colour:	Golden yellow
Aroma:	Sweet and delicate
Contraindications:	Avoid using on skin before exposure to sun as photosensitisation can occur.

GENERAL PROPERTIES:

Antiviral, relaxing, stimulant, uplifting

THERAPEUTIC PROPERTIES: (main uses underlined)

Circulatory:	Hypertension, palpitations
<u>*Digestive:*</u>	Colic, constipation, diarrhoea, flatulence, liver congestion, liver tonic, nausea, stomach tonic
Head:	Gingivitis
Muscular:	Cramp
Respiratory:	Hiccoughs
<u>*Skin:*</u>	Oily, regenerative, scars, stretchmarks

MARJORAM (Sweet)

Family:	Labiatae (Mint family)
Genus:	Origanum marjorana
	Note: Another variety of marjoram is

available – thymus mastichina (Spanish marjoram). Origanum marjorana, however, is the more highly recommended of the two.

Country of origin:	Hungary
Extraction:	Distilled from leaves and flowers
Volatility:	Middle note
Principal constituents:	Terpinene, terpineol, terpinen-4-ol, pinene
Colour:	Yellowish
Aroma:	Warm and spicy
Contraindications:	Do not use during the first six months of pregnancy.

GENERAL PROPERTIES:

Analgesic, antispasmodic, relaxing, sedative, tonic, warming

THERAPEUTIC PROPERTIES: (main uses underlined)

<u>*Circulatory:*</u>	Heart tonic, hypertension, low body temperature, poor circulation
Digestive:	Abdominal distension, air swallowing, colic, constipation, flatulence, indigestion, stimulates digestion
<u>*Emotional:*</u>	Anaphrodisiac, anxiety, exhaustion, grief, hysteria, insomnia, irritability, panic, run down, stress
Genito-urinary:	Leucorrhoea, menstruation – absent, scanty or painful periods
Head:	Headache, migraine
<u>*Muscular:*</u>	Aching, antispasmodic, arthritis, cramp, fibrositis, gout, rheumatism, rheumatoid arthritis, sprains, stiffness, strains
Neurological:	Nerve tonic, neuralgia, tic
<u>*Respiratory:*</u>	Asthma, bronchitis, catarrh, colds, coughs (tickly)
Skin:	Bruises, bunions, chilblains, wounds

MELISSA

Family:	Labiatae (Mint family)
Genus:	Melissa officinalis (lemon balm)
Country of origin:	France
Extraction:	Distilled from the whole plant
Volatility:	Middle note
Principal constituents:	Linaloöl, geraniol, citronellol, citral, citronellal
Colour:	Colourless to yellow
Aroma:	Musty and slightly sweet, lemony
Contraindications:	Use in low concentrations as it may cause irritation.
	Do not use during first five months of pregnancy.

GENERAL PROPERTIES:

Anti-allergic, anti-inflammatory, antispasmodic, antiviral, cooling, relaxing, sedative, tonic, uplifting

THERAPEUTIC PROPERTIES: (main uses underlined)

Circulatory:	Heart tonic, high body temperature, hypertension, palpitations
Digestive:	Abdominal distension, colic, dysentry, flatulence, gastritis, heartburn, indigestion, loss of appetite, nausea, stimulates digestion, stomach tonic, vomiting, worms
Emotional:	Anger, anxiety, depression, grief, hypersensitivity, hysteria, insomnia, irritability, panic, shock, stress
Genito-urinary:	Menopause, menstruation – absent, irregular, painful or scanty periods, PMS, sterility, uterine tonic
Head:	Alopecia, dizziness, fainting, halitosis, headache, migraine, vertigo
Muscular:	Antispasmodic

Neurological:	Nerve stimulant, nerve tonic, neuralgia, sciatica
Respiratory:	Asthma, bronchitis, catarrh, colds, hayfever
Skin:	Allergies, dermatitis, eczema, fevers, insect bites and stings, irritable, regenerative, sensitive

MYRRH

Family:	Burseraceae (Resinous trees and shrubs)
Genus:	Commiphora myrrha
Country of origin:	Europe
Extraction:	Distilled from resin (resinoid)
Volatility:	Base note
Principal constituents:	Pinene, dipentene, limonene, cadinene, formic acid, acetic acid, myrrholic acid, eugenol, aldehydes, alcohols and resins
Colour:	Yellow to red/brown
Aroma:	Musty and bitter
Contraindications:	Do not take internally. Do not use during pregnancy.

GENERAL PROPERTIES:

Anti-inflammatory, cooling, fungicidal, sedative, tonic

THERAPEUTIC PROPERTIES: (main uses underlined)

Circulatory:	Anaemia, high body temperature
Digestive:	Colic, diarrhoea, flatulence, haemorrhoids, indigestion, loss of appetite, stomach tonic
Emotional:	Insomnia
Genito-urinary:	Haemorrhage, leucorrhoea, menstruation – absent or painful periods, thrush, uterine tonic
Head:	Gingivitis, halitosis, laryngitis, loss of

voice, mouth ulcers, oral thrush, sore throat, stomatitis

Muscular:	Degeneration, wasting
Respiratory:	Asthma, bronchitis (chronic), catarrh, colds, coughs, diphtheria, tuberculosis
Skin:	Astringent, athlete's foot, blisters, boils, chapped, cracked, eczema (weeping), herpes, inflamed, mature, regenerative, ringworm, scars, stretchmarks, ulcers (weeping), wounds

MYRTLE

Family:	Myrtaceae (Shrubs and trees)
Genus:	Myrtus communis
Country of origin:	North Africa, Mediterranean
Extraction:	Distilled from leaves
Volatility:	Mid-base note
Principal constituents:	Myrtenol, cineol, pinene, geraniol
Colour:	Pale yellow
Aroma:	Camphoraceous
Contraindications:	Although this oil is considered mild enough for use with children, it should be treated, as all oils, as a potential irritant

GENERAL PROPERTIES:

Antiseptic, sedative

THERAPEUTIC PROPERTIES: (main uses underlined)

Circulatory:	Haemorrhoids
Emotional:	Insomnia
Genito-urinary:	Cystitis, urinary tract infections
Respiratory:	Bronchitis (chronic), catarrh, diphtheria, emphysema
Skin:	Acne, astringent, oily

n

NEROLI

Family:	Rutaceae (Citrus family)
Genus:	Citrus aurantium amara (bitter orange)
Country of origin:	Morocco
Extraction:	Distilled from flowers
Volatility:	Base note
Principal constituents:	Linalyl acetate (7 per cent), linaloöl (30 per cent), terpineol, nerol, geraniol and acetates (10 per cent), pinene, camphene, dipentene, paraffin (35 per cent)
Colour:	Yellowish
Aroma:	Bitter-sweet and musty
Contraindications:	Do not use in conjunction with chemotherapy in the treatment of cancer.

GENERAL PROPERTIES:

Antispasmodic, antiviral, detoxifying, relaxing, sedative, tonic, uplifting

THERAPEUTIC PROPERTIES: (main uses underlined)

Circulatory:	Blood purifier, heart tonic, hypertension, palpitations, poor circulation
Digestive:	Colitis, diarrhoea, flatulence, stimulates digestion
Emotional:	Anxiety, aphrodisiac, depression, fear, hysteria, insomnia, irritability, panic, paranoia, shock, stress
Genito-urinary:	Frigidity, impotence, PMS, sterility
Head:	Fainting
Muscular:	Antispasmodic

Skin:	Acne, allergies, broken capillaries, deodorant, dermatitis, eczema, irritable, mature, regenerative, scars, stretchmarks, supersensitive

NIAOULI

Family:	Myrtaceae (Shrubs and trees)
Genus:	Maleleuca viridiflora
Country of origin:	France
Extraction:	Distilled from leaves
Volatility:	Top note
Principal constituents:	Cineol (50–60 per cent), terpineol, pinene, benzaldehyde
Colour:	Yellow
Aroma:	Sweet and camphoraceous
Contraindications:	Although considered a mild oil, niaouli should still be regarded as a potential irritant

GENERAL PROPERTIES:

Analgesic, antiseptic (powerful), antiviral, fungicidal, stimulant

THERAPEUTIC PROPERTIES: (main uses underlined)

Circulatory:	Stimulates immune system
Digestive:	Colitis, diarrhoea, dysentry, gastroenteritis, indigestion, worms
Genito-urinary:	Cystitis, inflamed kidneys, kidney tonic, urinary tract infections
Head:	Deafness, earache, laryngitis, rhinitis, sinusitis, sore throat
Muscular:	Rheumatism
Respiratory:	Bronchitis (chronic), catarrh, colds, coughs, flu, pneumonia, whooping cough
Skin:	Acne, boils, burns, insect bites and stings, ulcers, wounds

O

ORANGE

Family:	Rutaceae (Citrus family)
Genus:	Citrus aurantium amara (bitter orange)
	Note: Oil of sweet orange (citrus aurantium sinensis) has similar therapeutic properties.
Country of origin:	Italy
Extraction:	Expressed from the peel of fruit
Volatility:	Top note
Principal constituents:	d-limonene (90 per cent), linalyl acetate, linaloöl, terpineol, citral
Colour:	Golden yellow
Aroma:	Sweet and warm
Contraindications:	Use in low concentrations as it may cause irritation or photosensitisation.

GENERAL PROPERTIES:

Antispasmodic, antiviral, relaxing, sedative, uplifting, warming

THERAPEUTIC PROPERTIES: (main uses underlined)

Circulatory:	Poor circulation
Digestive:	Colic, constipation, diarrhoea, flatulence, indigestion, travel sickness
Emotional:	Depression, insomnia
Genito-urinary:	Diuretic, fluid retention, menopause
Head:	Gingivitis, mouth ulcers
Muscular:	Antispasmodic
Respiratory:	Bronchitis, colds, hayfever
Skin:	Dry, irritable

p

PATCHOULI

Family:	Labiatae (Mint family)
Genus:	Pogostemon patchouli
Country of origin:	Indonesia
Extraction:	Distilled from leaves
Volatility:	Base note
Principal constituents:	Patchouli alcohol, terpenes, benzaldehyde, eugenol, cinnamic aldehyde
Colour:	Dark yellow to brown
Aroma:	Musty and heavy

GENERAL PROPERTIES:

Anti-inflammatory, antiviral, fungicidal, relaxing, stimulant, tonic, uplifting

THERAPEUTIC PROPERTIES: (main uses underlined)

Circulatory:	Lymphatic congestion, poor circulation
Digestive:	Constipation, diarrhoea
Emotional:	Anxiety, aphrodisiac, confusion, depression, indecision, stress
Genito-urinary:	Diuretic, fluid retention
Head:	Dandruff, seborrhoea of scalp
Neurological:	Nerve stimulant
Skin:	Acne, allergies, astringent, athlete's foot, burns, cellulite, chapped, cracked, deodorant, dermatitis, eczema (weeping), fevers, herpes, inflamed, insect bites and stings, insect repellent, mature, obesity, regenerative, scars, sensitive, sores (weeping), stretchmarks, tonic, wounds

PEPPERMINT

Family:	Labiatae (Mint family)
Genus:	Mentha piperita
Country of origin:	Mid-west America
Extraction:	Distilled from leaves and flowers
Volatility:	Middle note
Principal constituents:	Menthol (40–60 per cent), limonene, menthone, cadinene, phellandrene, pinene
Colour:	Colourless to pale yellow
Aroma:	Light and refreshing
Contraindications:	Use in low concentrations as it may cause irritation. Use in low concentrations during pregnancy. Do not use with epileptics.

GENERAL PROPERTIES:

Analgesic, antiseptic (powerful), antispasmodic, antiviral, cooling, fungicidal, stimulant, tonic, uplifting

THERAPEUTIC PROPERTIES: (main uses underlined)

Circulatory:	Anaemia, heart tonic, high body temperature, hypotension, palpitations, varicose veins, vasoconstrictor
Digestive:	Abdominal distension, acid stomach, air swallowing, cholera, colic, colitis, diarrhoea, flatulence, food poisoning, gall stones, gastralgia, gastroenteritis, haemorrhoids, heartburn, indigestion, liver tonic, nausea, stimulates digestion, stomach tonic, travel sickness, ulcers, vomiting, worms
Emotional:	Confusion, depression, exhaustion, hysteria, indecision, insomnia, irritability, panic, poor concentration or memory, run down, shock

Genito-urinary:	Impotence, menopause, menstruation – absent, irregular, painful or scanty periods, sterility, vaginal irritation
Glandular:	Decreases flow of breast milk, mastitis
Head:	Dizziness, earache, fainting, halitosis, headache, migraine, sinusitis, sore throat, toothache, vertigo
Muscular:	Antispasmodic, arthritis, gout
Neurological:	Nerve tonic, neuralgia, paralysis
Respiratory:	Asthma, bronchitis (chronic), catarrh, colds, coughs, flu, pneumonia, tuberculosis
Skin:	Acne, astringent, athlete's foot, broken capillaries, bruises, bunions, congested, dermatitis, eczema, fevers, inflamed, insect repellent, irritable, lice, ringworm, scabies, shingles

PETITGRAIN

Family:	Rutaceae (Citrus family)
Genus:	Citrus aurantium amara (bitter orange)
Country of origin:	Paraguay
Extraction:	Distilled from leaves
Volatility:	Top note
Principal constituents:	Linaloöl (40 per cent), linalyl acetate (50 per cent)
Colour:	Colourless
Aroma:	Sweet and musty

GENERAL PROPERTIES:

Antiviral, relaxing, stimulant, uplifting

THERAPEUTIC PROPERTIES: (main uses underlined)

Circulatory:	Swollen lymph nodes
Emotional:	Anxiety, depression, stress

Genito-urinary:	Diuretic, fluid retention
Neurological:	Nerve tonic
Skin:	Acne, deodorant

PINE (Needle)

Family:	Pinaceae (Conifer family)
Genus:	Pinus sylvestris
Country of origin:	Spain
Extraction:	Distilled from needles
Volatility:	Middle note
Principal constituents:	Bornyl acetate, borneol
Colour:	Pale yellow
Aroma:	Fresh and light
Contraindications:	Use in low concentrations as it may cause irritation.

GENERAL PROPERTIES:

Analgesic, antiseptic (powerful), antispasmodic, stimulant, uplifting

THERAPEUTIC PROPERTIES: (main uses underlined)

Circulatory:	Anaemia, haemorrhage, inflamed lymph nodes, poor circulation, stimulates production of white blood cells
Digestive:	Abdominal distension, colic, gallstones, gastralgia, gastroenteritis, liver tonic, worms
Emotional:	Bedwetting, exhaustion, poor concentration or memory, run down
Genito-urinary:	Cystitis, impotence, incontinence, inflamed kidneys, intramenstrual bleeding, kidney tonic, leucorrhoea, menopause, menstrual pain, urinary tract infections
Glandular:	Prostatitis, stimulates adrenal cortex

Head:	Migraine, nosebleed, sinusitis, sore throat
Muscular:	Aching, antispasmodic, arthritis, fibrositis, gout, rheumatism, rheumatoid arthritis, rickets
Neurological:	Neuralgia, sciatica
Respiratory:	Asthma, bronchitis (chronic), catarrh, colds, coughs (convulsive), flu, haemoptysis, hayfever, pneumonia
Skin:	Deodorant, fever, lice, wounds

r

ROSE

Family:	Rosaceae (Rose family)
Genus:	Rosa centifolia (cabbage rose)
	Rosa damascena (damask rose)
	Note: Distilled rose oil is known as Rose Otto. It is a more expensive oil but reputedly of even greater therapeutic value than the absolute.
Country of origin:	Bulgaria
Extraction:	An absolute extracted from flowers by enfleurage
Volatility:	Base note
Principal constituents:	Phenylethyl alcohol (60–70 per cent), citronellol (20 per cent), geraniol and nerol (13 per cent)
Colour:	Yellow/brown (cabbage rose), red/brown (damask rose)
Aroma:	Sweet and floral
Contraindications:	Do not take absolute internally. Although rose is considered one of the least toxic oils it should not be used by pregnant women because of its powerful emmenagogic effect (it induces menstruation), nor should it be used in conjunction with chemotherapy in the treatment of cancer.

GENERAL PROPERTIES:

Antispasmodic, cooling, detoxifying, haemostatic, relaxing, sedative, tonic

THERAPEUTIC PROPERTIES: (main uses underlined)

Circulatory:	Blood purifier, haemorrhage, heart tonic,

high body temperature, palpitations, poor circulation, spleen tonic, vasoconstrictor

Digestive: Constipation, liver tonic, nausea, stomach tonic, ulcers, vomiting

Emotional: Anger, anorexia, anxiety, aphrodisiac, depression, grief, hysteria, insomnia, irritability, jealousy, panic, shock, stress

Genito-urinary: Frigidity, haemorrhage, impotence, leucorrhoea, menopause, menstruation – absent, heavy, irregular or scanty periods, PMS, sterility, uterine tonic

Head: Conjunctivitis, earache, headache, migraine

Muscular: Antispasmodic

Respiratory: Coughs (tickly), hayfever

Skin: Acne, allergies, astringent, boils, broken capillaries, carbuncles, chapped, cracked, dermatitis, dry, eczema, inflamed, mature, regenerative, scars, stretchmarks, supersensitive, thread veins, wounds

ROSEMARY

Family: Labiatae (Mint family)
Genus: Rosmarinus officinalis
Country of origin: Italy
Extraction: Distilled from the whole plant
Volatility: Middle note
Principal constituents: Cineol, borneol, pinene, camphene, camphor, dipentene, caryophyllene
Colour: Colourless
Aroma: Fresh, sweet and camphoraceous
Contraindications: Use in low concentrations.

Do not use in the first five months of pregnancy.
Do not use with hypertensives.

GENERAL PROPERTIES:

Analgesic, antiseptic (powerful), antispasmodic, antiviral, stimulant, tonic, uplifting, warming

THERAPEUTIC PROPERTIES: (main uses underlined)

Circulatory:	Anaemia, arteriosclerosis, heart tonic, high blood cholesterol, hypotension, inflamed lymph nodes, low body temperature, lymphatic congestion, palpitations, poor circulation, varicose veins
Digestive:	Abdominal distension, colic, colitis, constipation, diarrhoea, flatulence, gall stones, gastralgia, gastroenteritis, hepatitis, indigestion, intestinal infections, jaundice, liver cirrhosis, liver congestion, liver tonic, stimulates digestion, stomach tonic, ulcers, vomiting
Emotional:	Anxiety, confusion, exhaustion, hysteria, indecision, panic, poor concentration or memory, run down, stress
Genito-urinary:	Diuretic, fluid retention, impotence, inflamed uterus, leucorrhoea, menopause, menstruation – absent, painful or scanty periods, PMS
Glandular:	Diabetes, stimulates adrenal cortex
Head:	Alopecia, dandruff, dizziness, earache, fainting, halitosis, headache, loss of sense of smell, loss of speech, migraine, oral thrush, sinusitis, sore throat, tonsillitis, vertigo, weak eyesight
Muscular:	Aching, antispasmodic, arthritis, fibrositis, gout, lack of tone, rheumatism,

rheumatoid arthritis, rickets, sprains, stiffness, strains

Neurological: Epilepsy, nerve stimulant, nerve tonic, neuralgia, paralysis

Respiratory: Asthma, bronchitis (chronic), catarrh, colds, coughs, flu, tuberculosis, whooping cough

Skin: Astringent, bruises, burns, cellulite, congested, fevers, lice, obesity, oily, scabies, sores, wounds

ROSEWOOD

Family:	Lauraceae (Laurel family)
Genus:	Aniba roseadora
Country of origin:	Brazil
Extraction:	Distilled from wood
Volatility:	Middle note
Principal constituents:	Linaloöl (80–90 per cent), terpineol, nerol, geraniol
Colour:	Pale yellow
Aroma:	Floral, musty, slightly citrus
Contraindications:	Not really known, but considered to be an especially toxic oil.

GENERAL PROPERTIES:

Analgesic (mild), relaxing, tonic, uplifting

THERAPEUTIC PROPERTIES: (main uses underlined)

Emotional: Aphrodisiac, confusion, depression, fear, panic, irritability

Head: Headache

Skin: Deodorant

S

SAGE

Family:	Labiatae (Mint family)
Genus:	Salvia officinalis
Country of origin:	France
Extraction:	Distilled from leaves
Volatility:	Top note
Principal constituents:	Thujone (40–60 per cent), borneol (10–15 per cent), bornyl acetate, salvene, pinene, cineole, and camphor
Colour:	Colourless
Aroma:	Woody and camphoraceous
Contraindications:	Use only under the guidance of a professional aromatherapist. Do not use with epileptics, hypertensives or during the first eight months of pregnancy. Use **Clary-sage** as a less toxic alternative.

GENERAL PROPERTIES:

Analgesic, anti-cancer, antispasmodic, haemostatic, stimulant, tonic, warming

THERAPEUTIC PROPERTIES: (main uses underlined)

Circulatory:	Haemorrhage, hypotension, inflamed lymph nodes, low body temperature, lymphatic congestion, varicose veins
Digestive:	Constipation, diarrhoea, flatulence, indigestion, intestinal infections, liver tonic, loss of appetite, stimulates digestion, stomach tonic
Emotional:	Exhaustion, irritability, poor concentration or memory, run down

Genito-urinary:	Diuretic, fluid retention, haemorrhage, inflamed uterus, kidney tonic, leucorrhoea, menopause, menstruation – absent, heavy, painful or scanty periods, ovarian tonic, sterility, thrush, urinary tract infections
Glandular:	Decreases flow of breast milk, stimulates adrenal cortex
Head:	Alopecia, dizziness, gingivitis, glossitis, headache, laryngitis, mouth ulcers, oral thrush, sore throat, stomatitis, tonsillitis, toothache, weak gums
Muscular:	Aching, antispasmodic, arthritis, fibrositis, gout, rheumatism, rheumatoid arthritis, sprains
Neurological:	Nerve tonic, paralysis
Respiratory:	Asthma, bronchitis (chronic), flu
Skin:	Animal bites, astringent, bruises, burns, congested, deodorant, dermatitis, eczema, insect bites and stings, sweating, tonic, ulcers, wounds

SANDALWOOD

Family:	Santalaceae (Sandalwood family)
Genus:	Santalum album
Country of origin:	India
Extraction:	Distilled from the heartwood
Volatility:	Base note
Principal constituents:	Santalol (over 90 per cent), santalene, santalone, santene, santenone, santenol, acids and aldehydes
Colour:	Yellow/brown
Aroma:	Sweet, spicy and woody

GENERAL PROPERTIES:

Antispasmodic, relaxing, sedative, tonic

THERAPEUTIC PROPERTIES: (main uses underlined)

Circulatory:	Heart tonic, stimulates production of white blood cells, varicose veins
Digestive:	Colic, diarrhoea, gastritis, haemorrhoids, heartburn, nausea, vomiting
Emotional:	Anxiety, aphrodisiac, depression, insomnia, stress
Genito-urinary:	Cystitis, diuretic, fluid retention, frigidity, gonorrhoea, impotence, kidney tonic, leucorrhoea, menopause, PMS, urinary tract infections
Glandular:	Balances female sex hormones
Head:	Dandruff, laryngitis, sore throat
Muscular:	Antispasmodic
Respiratory:	Asthma, bronchitis (chronic), catarrh, cough (dry or painful), flu, hiccoughs, tuberculosis
Skin:	Acne, allergies, astringent, chapped, cracked, dry, eczema, inflamed, irritable, mature, oily, sores, sunburn

t

TAGETES (Marigold)

Family:	Compositae (Daisy family)
Genus:	Tagetes glandulifera
Country of origin:	Africa
Extraction:	Distilled from flowers
Volatility:	Base note
Principal constituents:	Tagetone (50–60 per cent), other ketones (5–10 per cent), limonene and ocymene
Colour:	Yellow/red
Aroma:	Heavy, pungent and sweet
Contraindications:	Do not take internally.

GENERAL PROPERTIES:

Fungicidal

THERAPEUTIC PROPERTIES: (main uses underlined)

<u>*Skin:*</u>	Athlete's foot, fungal conditions of the nails, psoriasis, ringworm

TEA-TREE (Ti-tree)

Family:	Myrtaceae (Shrubs and trees)
Genus:	Maleleuca alternifolia
Country of origin:	Australia
Extraction:	Distilled from leaves
Volatility:	Top note
Principal constituents:	Pinene, cymene, cineole, terpenes, terpinene, alcohols
Colour:	Colourless to pale yellow
Aroma:	Pungent and stale
Contraindications:	Use in low concentrations as it may cause irritation.

GENERAL PROPERTIES:

Anti-cancer, antiseptic (powerful), antiviral, cooling, fungicidal, tonic

THERAPEUTIC PROPERTIES: (main uses underlined)

Circulatory:	Stimulates immune system
Digestive:	Colitis, diarrhoea, gastroenteritis, indigestion
Genito-urinary:	Cystitis, inflamed kidneys, thrush, urinary tract infections
Glandular:	Glandular fever
Head:	Gingivitis, mouth ulcers, oral thrush, sinusitis, sore throat, stomatitis, tonsillitis
Respiratory:	Bronchitis, catarrh, colds, flu, pneumonia, whooping cough
Skin:	Abscess, acne, athlete's foot, boils, chicken pox, corns, fevers, herpes, inflamed, insect bites and stings, lice, measles, regenerative, ringworm, scars, shingles, snakebite, stretchmarks, sunburn, sores, verrucae, warts, wounds

THYME

Family:	Labiatae (Mint family)
Genus:	Thymus vulgaris
Country of origin:	France
Extraction:	Distilled from flowers
Volatility:	Middle note
Principal constituents:	Thymol and carvacrol (60 per cent)
Colour:	Colourless
Aroma:	Light, fresh and slightly musty
Contraindications:	Use only under the guidance of a professional aromatherapist. Do not use with children, hypertensives or during pregnancy.

GENERAL PROPERTIES:

Antiseptic (powerful), antispasmodic, antiviral, sedative, tonic, warming

THERAPEUTIC PROPERTIES: (main uses underlined)

Circulatory:	Anaemia, hypotension, low body temperature, palpitations, poor circulation, stimulates production of white blood cells
Digestive:	Colitis, dysentry, flatulence, gastroenteritis, indigestion, intestinal infections, liver congestion, liver tonic, loss of appetite, stimulates digestion, worms
Emotional:	Anxiety, confusion, exhaustion, hysteria, indecision, panic, poor concentration or memory, run down, stress
Genito-urinary:	Cystitis, diuretic, fluid retention, inflamed kidneys, inflamed uterus, kidney tonic, leucorrhoea, menstruation – absent or scanty periods, urinary tract infections, vaginal irritation, vaginitis
Head:	Alopecia, dizziness, gingivitis, halitosis, headache, laryngitis, mumps, oral thrush, quinsy, rhinitis, sinusitis, sore throat, tonsillitis, toothache, weak gums
Muscular:	Aching, antispasmodic, arthritis, fibrositis, gout, rheumatism, rheumatoid arthritis, rickets, sprains, stiffness
Neurological:	Nerve tonic
Respiratory:	Asthma, bronchitis, catarrh, colds, coughs (convulsive), emphysema, flu, whooping cough
Skin:	Boils, deodorant, fevers, insect bites and stings, lice, measles, scabies, snakebite, sores, wounds

Y

YLANG-YLANG

Family:	Annonaceae (Magnolia family)
Genus:	Cananga odorata
Country of origin:	Réunion
Extraction:	Distilled from flowers
Volatility:	Base note
Principal constituents:	Geraniol, linaloöl, cadinene, pinene, eugenol, eugenol methyl ether, methyl anthranilate, methyl benzoate, methyl salicylate, benzyl benzoate, benzyl acetate, iso-safrole, alcohols and esters (50–60 per cent), sesquiterpenes (35 per cent)
Colour:	Colourless to pale yellow
Aroma:	Heavy, sweet, floral
Contraindications:	May cause headache or nausea in high concentrations.

GENERAL PROPERTIES:

Relaxing, sedative, uplifting

THERAPEUTIC PROPERTIES: (main uses underlined)

Circulatory:	Hypertension, palpitations
Digestive:	Colitis, gall stones, gastroenteritis, intestinal infections
Emotional:	Anger, anxiety, aphrodisiac, depression, hysteria, insomnia, irritability, panic, stress
Genito-urinary:	Frigidity, impotence
Head:	Alopecia
Neurological:	Nerve tonic
Respiratory:	Deep and rapid breathing
Skin:	Dry, insect bites and stings, oily, sores

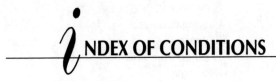

INDEX OF CONDITIONS

Please note: those oils which are *italicised* are especially useful for the condition; oils in brackets are relatively toxic and should be reserved for acute conditions only.

GENERAL PROPERTIES OF ESSENTIAL OILS

Analgesic – pain relieving:
Bergamot, black pepper, cajeput, (camphor), chamomile, (clove), coriander, *eucalyptus*, geranium, *juniper*, *lavender*, *marjoram*, niaouli, peppermint, pine, *rosemary*, rosewood, (sage).

Anti-allergic – reduces allergic reaction:
Chamomile, melissa.

Anti-cancer – helpful in relief of symptoms:
Bergamot, cedarwood, *chamomile*, (clove), cypress, *eucalyptus*, garlic, geranium, (hyssop), *lavender*, (sage), tea-tree.
(NB Avoid massage in treating cancers, especially Hodgkins disease or bone cancers.)

Anti-inflammatory – reduces inflammation:
Bergamot, calendula, *chamomile*, clary-sage, geranium, *lavender*, melissa, myrrh, patchouli.

Antiseptic:
All oils are antiseptic. The most powerful however are:
Bergamot, (cajeput), (cinnamon), (clove), *eucalyptus*, garlic, *juniper*, *lavender*, *lemon*, (lemongrass), myrtle, niaouli, peppermint, pine, *rosemary*, tea-tree, (thyme).

Antispasmodic – relieves smooth muscle spasm:
Basil, bergamot, black pepper, (cajeput), (camphor), caraway, cardamom, *chamomile*, clary-sage, (clove), coriander, cypress, *eucalyptus*, fennel, (hyssop), jasmine, *juniper*, *lavender*, *marjoram*, melissa, neroli, orange, peppermint, rose, *rosemary*, (sage), sandalwood, (thyme).

Antiviral – effective against viruses:
Bergamot, (cajeput), clary-sage, (clove), *eucalyptus*, garlic, hyssop, *juniper*, *lavender*, *lemon*, mandarin, melissa, neroli, niaouli, orange, patchouli, peppermint, petitgrain, *rosemary*, tea-tree, (thyme).

Balancing – balances mind and body:
(Camphor), cedarwood, geranium, *juniper*, *lavender*.

Cooling:
Bergamot, cypress, *eucalyptus, lavender*, melissa, myrrh, peppermint, rose, tea-tree.

Detoxifying – counteracts toxins in general:
Black pepper, cedarwood, (cinnamon), *eucalyptus*, fennel, garlic, *juniper, lavender, lemon*, neroli, rose.
NB **Do not** use these oils in conjunction with chemotherapy in the treatment of cancer.

Fungicidal – effective against fungal infections:
(Cajeput), calendula, garlic, *lavender, lemon*, myrrh, niaouli, patchouli, peppermint, tagetes, tea-tree.

Haemostatic – stops bleeding:
(Cinnamon), cypress, *eucalyptus*, frankincense, geranium, *lemon*, rose, (sage). (Use lemon as first aid for cuts.)

Relaxing:
Benzoin, bergamot, *chamomile*, clary-sage, cypress, frankincense, geranium, (hyssop), jasmine, *juniper, lavender*, mandarin, *marjoram*, melissa, neroli, orange, patchouli, petitgrain, rose, rosewood, sandalwood, ylang-ylang.

Sedative:
Benzoin, bergamot, (camphor), cedarwood, *chamomile*, clary-sage, cypress, frankincense, geranium, jasmine, *juniper*, lavender, *marjoram*, melissa, myrrh, myrtle, neroli, rose, sandalwood, (thyme), ylang-ylang.

Stimulant:
Basil, black pepper, (cajeput), (camphor), caraway, cardamom, (cinnamon), (clove), coriander, *eucalyptus*, geranium, (hyssop), *juniper, lemon*, (lemongrass), mandarin, niaouli, patchouli, peppermint, petitgrain, pine, *rosemary*, (sage).

Tonic:
Basil, black pepper, cardamom, *chamomile*, (cinnamon), clary-sage, (clove), cypress, fennel, frankincense, geranium, grapefruit, (hyssop), jasmine, *juniper, lavender, lemon*, (lemongrass), *marjoram*, melissa, myrrh, neroli, patchouli, peppermint, rose, *rosemary*, rosewood, (sage), sandalwood, tea-tree, (thyme).

Uplifting:
Basil, bergamot, cardamom, *chamomile*, clary-sage, cypress, *eucalyptus*, frankincense, geranium, grapefruit, jasmine, *juniper*, *lavender*, *lemon*, (lemongrass), mandarin, melissa, neroli, orange, patchouli, peppermint, petitgrain, pine, *rosemary*, rosewood, ylang-ylang.

Warming:
Basil, benzoin, black pepper, (cajeput), (camphor), caraway, cardamom, (cinnamon), clary-sage, (clove), coriander, fennel, frankincense, geranium, ginger, jasmine, *juniper*, *marjoram*, orange, *rosemary*, (sage), (thyme).

CIRCULATORY RELATED CONDITIONS

Alcohol poisoning:
Fennel.

Anaemia:
Black pepper, chamomile, garlic, lavender, lemon, myrrh, peppermint, pine, *rosemary*, (*thyme*).

Angina – suffocating chest pain:
Black pepper.

Arteriosclerosis – hardening of artery walls:
Garlic, juniper, lemon, rosemary.

Blood cholesterol – high:
Garlic, juniper, rosemary.

Blood purifying oils:
Cedarwood, *cypress*, eucalyptus, *fennel*, grapefruit, *juniper*, *lemon*, neroli, rose.

Blood sugar - high:
Eucalyptus, geranium, *juniper*.

Body temperature – high:
Bergamot, *cypress*, eucalyptus, *lavender*, *melissa*, myrrh, peppermint, rose.

Body temperature – low:
Benzoin, *black pepper*, (camphor), caraway, cardamom, (cinnamon), ginger, *juniper*, *marjoram*, *rosemary*, (sage), (*thyme*).

Haemorrhage:
(Cinnamon), *cypress*, eucalyptus, frankincense, geranium, *juniper*, *lemon*, pine, rose, (sage).

Heart tonic:
Benzoin, (camphor), *garlic*, (hyssop), *lavender*, *lemon*, marjoram, *melissa*.

Hypertension – high blood pressure:
Clary-sage, garlic, juniper, lavender, lemon, marjoram, *melissa*, neroli, (sage), *ylang-ylang*.

Hypotension – low blood pressure:
Black pepper, (camphor), (cinnamon), (hyssop), *lemon*, peppermint, *rosemary*, (sage), (*thyme*).

Immune system stimulant:
(Cajeput), *garlic*, lavender, niaouli, tea-tree.

Lymphatic congestion:
Black pepper, cedarwood, *fennel*, geranium, *juniper*, lavender, patchouli, *rosemary*, (sage).

Lymph nodes swollen or inflamed:
Caraway, (clove), *garlic*, lavender, petitgrain, pine, *rosemary*, (sage).

Malaria – an infectious disease caused by a parasite:
Basil, eucalyptus, *garlic*, lemon.

Palpitations:
Chamomile, eucalyptus, *garlic*, lavender, mandarin, *melissa*, neroli, peppermint, rose, *rosemary*, (*thyme*), ylang-ylang.

Poor circulation:
Benzoin, *black pepper*, (cajeput), (camphor), caraway, cardamom, (cinnamon), (clove), coriander, *cypress*, eucalyptus, *garlic*, geranium, ginger, *juniper*, lavender, lemon, (lemongrass), marjoram, neroli, orange, patchouli, pine, rose, *rosemary*, (*thyme*).

Spleen tonic:
Black pepper, chamomile, fennel, juniper, lavender, rose.

Varicose veins:
Calendula, cypress, garlic, juniper, lavender, lemon, peppermint, *rosemary*, (sage), sandalwood.

Vasoconstrictor – narrows blood vessels:
(Camphor), chamomile, cypress, peppermint, rose.

White blood cell stimulant:
All essential oils stimulate production of white blood cells. The most useful however are:
Bergamot, chamomile, lavender, lemon, pine, sandalwood, (thyme).

DIGESTIVE RELATED CONDITIONS

Abdominal distension:
Caraway, chamomile, (cinnamon), (clove), coriander, fennel, garlic, ginger, (hyssop), lavender, marjoram, melissa, peppermint, pine, rosemary

Acid stomach:
Black pepper, (cinnamon), (clove), lemon, peppermint.

Air swallowing:
Caraway, coriander, lemon, marjoram, peppermint.

Cholera – acute bacterial infection of the small intestine:
Black pepper, (camphor), (cinnamon), eucalyptus, juniper, peppermint.

Colic – waves of abdominal pain:
Basil, benzoin, bergamot, black pepper, (camphor), caraway, cardamom, chamomile, (cinnamon), clary-sage, coriander, fennel, frankincense, garlic, ginger, (hyssop), juniper, lavender, lemon, mandarin, marjoram, melissa, myrrh, orange, peppermint, pine, rosemary, sandalwood.

Colitis – inflammation of the colon:
Bergamot, black pepper, (cajeput), chamomile, coriander, fennel, garlic, (hyssop), juniper, lavender, (lemongrass), neroli, niaouli, peppermint, rosemary, tea-tree, (thyme), ylang-ylang.

Constipation:
Black pepper, (camphor), chamomile, (cinnamon), fennel, ginger, grapefruit, (hyssop), lemon, mandarin, marjoram, orange, patchouli, rose, rosemary, (sage).

Diarrhoea:
Black pepper, (camphor), *chamomile*, (cinnamon), (clove),
cypress, eucalyptus, *garlic*, geranium, *ginger*, *juniper*, *lavender*,
lemon, *mandarin*, myrrh, neroli, niaouli, *orange*, patchouli,
peppermint, rosemary, (sage), sandalwood, tea-tree.

Digestive stimulant:
Basil, bergamot, *black pepper*, (camphor), caraway, *cardamom*,
chamomile, (cinnamon), clary-sage, *coriander*, *fennel*,
frankincense, *garlic*, *ginger*, grapefruit, (hyssop), (lemongrass),
juniper, marjoram, melissa, neroli, *peppermint*, rosemary,
(sage), (*thyme*).

Dysentry – intestinal infection caused by amoeba or bacteria:
Basil, *black pepper*, (cajeput), *chamomile*, cypress, eucalyptus,
garlic, *juniper*, lemon, melissa, niaouli, (*thyme*).

Flatulence:
Basil, bergamot, *black pepper*, (camphor), caraway, *cardamom*,
chamomile, (cinnamon), clary-sage, (clove), *coriander*, *fennel*,
ginger, (hyssop), *juniper*, *lavender*, *lemon*, *mandarin*,
marjoram, melissa, myrrh, neroli, *orange*, *peppermint*,
rosemary, (sage), (*thyme*).

Food poisoning:
Black pepper, fennel, *peppermint*.

Gall stones:
Bergamot, (camphor), *chamomile*, eucalyptus, *garlic*, geranium,
(hyssop), *lavender*, *lemon*, *peppermint*, pine, rosemary, ylang-
ylang.

Gastralgia – stomach pain:
Bergamot, *chamomile*, (cinnamon), *coriander*, fennel, garlic,
geranium, (hyssop), *lavender*, *peppermint*, pine, rosemary.

Gastritis – inflammation of the stomach lining:
(Cajeput), calendula, caraway, *chamomile*, lemon, melissa,
sandalwood.

Gastroenteritis – inflammation of the stomach and intestine:
Basil, bergamot, (cajeput), calendula, (camphor), *chamomile*,
garlic, geranium, (hyssop), *lavender*, (lemongrass), niaouli,
peppermint, pine, rosemary, tea-tree, (*thyme*), ylang-ylang.

Haemorrhoids (piles) – enlarged veins in the wall of the anus:
Calendula, cypress, frankincense, garlic, geranium, juniper, myrrh, myrtle, peppermint, sandalwood.

Heartburn – pain behind the breastbone:
Black pepper, cardamom, lemon, melissa, peppermint, sandalwood.

Hepatitis – inflammation of the liver:
Rosemary.

Indigestion – pain in abdomen and lower chest after eating:
Basil, bergamot, black pepper, (cajeput), calendula, caraway, cardamom, chamomile, (cinnamon), clary-sage, (clove), coriander, eucalyptus, fennel, frankincense, garlic, ginger, (hyssop), juniper, lavender, lemon, (lemongrass), marjoram, melissa, myrrh, niaouli, orange, peppermint, rosemary, (sage).

Intestinal infections:
Basil, garlic, rosemary, (sage), (thyme), ylang-ylang.

Jaundice – excess bile pigments in the blood:
Chamomile, geranium, lemon, rosemary.

Liver - cirrhosis:
Juniper, rosemary.

Liver - congested:
Chamomile, cypress, lemon, mandarin, rosemary, (thyme).

Liver tonic:
Calendula, chamomile, cypress, geranium, grapefruit, lemon, mandarin, peppermint, pine, rose, rosemary, (sage), (thyme).

Loss of appetite:
Basil, bergamot, black pepper, caraway, cardamom, chamomile, (cinnamon), coriander, fennel, ginger, (hyssop), juniper, lavender, lemon, melissa, myrrh, (sage), (thyme).

Nausea:
Basil, black pepper, caraway, cardamom, (clove), fennel, ginger, lavender, mandarin, melissa, peppermint, rose, sandalwood.

Stomach tonic:
Basil, black pepper, caraway, cardamom, chamomile, clary-sage, (clove), coriander, fennel, grapefruit, juniper, mandarin, melissa, myrrh, peppermint, rose, rosemary, (sage).

Travel sickness:
Ginger, lavender, orange, peppermint.

Typhoid – bacterial infection of the digestive system:
Eucalyptus, garlic, juniper, lavender, lemon.

Ulcers:
Calendula, chamomile, garlic, geranium, lavender, lemon, peppermint, rose, rosemary.

Vomiting:
Basil, black pepper, (cajeput), (camphor), cardamom, chamomile, fennel, lavender, lemon, melissa, peppermint, rose, rosemary, sandalwood.

Worms:
Bergamot, (cajeput), (camphor), caraway, chamomile, (cinnamon), (clove), eucalyptus, fennel, garlic, (hyssop), lavender, melissa, peppermint, pine, (thyme).

EMOTIONAL CONDITIONS

The individual's preference for aromas is doubly important when choosing essential oils to help an emotional problem as aromas have different associations for different people.

Anaphrodisiac – reduces sexual excitement:
Marjoram.

Anger:
Chamomile, melissa, rose, ylang-ylang.

Anorexia:
Bergamot, coriander, jasmine, rose.

Anxiety/stress:
Basil, benzoin, bergamot, calendula, (camphor), cedarwood, chamomile, clary-sage, cypress, frankincense, geranium, jasmine, juniper, lavender, (lemongrass), marjoram, melissa, neroli, patchouli, petitgrain, rose, sandalwood, (thyme), ylang-ylang.

Aphrodisiac:
Black pepper, cardamom, clary-sage, jasmine, juniper, neroli, patchouli, rose, rosewood, sandalwood, ylang-ylang.

Bedwetting:
Cypress, pine.

Confusion/indecision:
Basil, cypress, eucalyptus, frankincense, geranium, patchouli, *peppermint*, *rosemary*, rosewood.

Depression:
Basil, bergamot, (camphor), *chamomile*, (cinnamon), *clary-sage*, coriander, eucalyptus, frankincense, geranium, ginger, grapefruit, *jasmine*, *lavender*, lemon, melissa, *neroli*, orange, patchouli, *peppermint*, petitgrain, *rose*, rosewood, sandalwood, (thyme), *ylang-ylang*.

Exhaustion:
Basil, *benzoin*, cardamom, (cinnamon), *clary-sage*, (clove), coriander, eucalyptus, geranium, *lavender*, lemon, *marjoram*, *peppermint*, pine, *rosemary*, (sage), (thyme).

Fear/paranoia:
Basil, *chamomile*, *clary-sage*, frankincense, *jasmine*, juniper, *neroli*, rosewood.

Grief:
Benzoin, cypress, (hyssop), *marjoram*, melissa, *rose*.

Hypersensitivity:
Chamomile, geranium, *jasmine*, melissa.

Hysteria/panic:
Basil, *benzoin*, bergamot, (camphor), cedarwood, *chamomile*, *clary-sage*, frankincense, geranium, *jasmine*, juniper, *lavender*, (lemongrass), *marjoram*, melissa, *neroli*, peppermint, *rose*, *rosemary*, rosewood, (thyme), *ylang-ylang*.

Insomnia:
Basil, *benzoin*, bergamot, (camphor), cedarwood, *chamomile*, *clary-sage*, cypress, frankincense, geranium, jasmine, juniper, *lavender*, *marjoram*, melissa, myrrh, myrtle, *neroli*, orange, *peppermint*, *rose*, sandalwood, (thyme), *ylang-ylang*.

Irritability/impatience:
(Camphor), caraway, *chamomile*, *clary-sage*, cypress, frankincense, *lavender*, *marjoram*, melissa, *neroli*, *peppermint*, *rose*, rosewood, (sage), *ylang-ylang*.

Jealousy:
Benzoin, chamomile, rose.

Poor memory/concentration:
Basil, cardamom, (cinnamon), (clove), coriander, geranium, (hyssop), lavender, peppermint, pine, rosemary, (sage), (thyme).

Run down:
Basil, benzoin, (camphor), cardamom, (cinnamon), clary-sage, (clove), coriander, eucalyptus, garlic, geranium, ginger, grapefruit, (hyssop), jasmine, juniper, lavender, lemon, marjoram, peppermint, pine, rosemary, (sage), (thyme).

Shock:
Basil, (camphor), cedarwood, chamomile, geranium, lavender, melissa, neroli, peppermint, rose.

GENITO-URINARY CONDITIONS

Cystitis – inflammation of the bladder:
Benzoin, bergamot, black pepper, (cajeput), cedarwood, chamomile, eucalyptus, fennel, frankincense, garlic, juniper, lavender, myrtle, niaouli, pine, sandalwood, tea-tree, (thyme).

Diuretic/fluid retention – encourages fluid loss by increasing urination:
Benzoin, bergamot, black pepper, (camphor), caraway, cardamom, cedarwood, chamomile, clary-sage, cypress, eucalyptus, fennel, frankincense, geranium, grapefruit, (hyssop), juniper, lavender, lemon, orange, patchouli, petitgrain, rosemary, (sage), sandalwood, (thyme).

Frigidity:
Clary-sage, geranium, jasmine, neroli, rose, sandalwood, ylang-ylang.

Gonorrhoea:
Bergamot, cedarwood, eucalyptus, frankincense, jasmine, lavender, lemon, sandalwood.

Impotence:
(Cinnamon), clary-sage, (clove), geranium, jasmine, neroli, peppermint, pine, rose, rosemary, sandalwood, ylang-ylang.

Incontinence – involuntary passing of urine:
Cypress, pine.

Kidneys – inflamed:
Cedarwood, chamomile, eucalyptus, frankincense, geranium, juniper, niaouli, pine, tea-tree, (thyme).

Kidney stones:
Chamomile, fennel, garlic, geranium, (hyssop), juniper, lemon.

Kidney tonic:
Cedarwood, chamomile, clary-sage, eucalyptus, fennel, geranium, grapefruit, juniper, lavender, lemon, niaouli, pine, (sage), sandalwood, (thyme).

Leucorrhoea – white/yellow vaginal discharge:
Benzoin, bergamot, cedarwood, (cinnamon), clary-sage, eucalyptus, frankincense, geranium, (hyssop), juniper, lavender, marjoram, myrrh, pine, rose, rosemary, (sage), sandalwood, (thyme).

Menopause:
Calendula, chamomile, clary-sage, cypress, fennel, geranium, jasmine, lavender, lemon, melissa, orange, peppermint, pine, rose, rosemary, (sage), sandalwood.

Menstruation:

Amenorrhoea – absence of periods:
Basil, chamomile, clary-sage, (clove), fennel, (hyssop), juniper, lavender, marjoram, melissa, myrrh, peppermint, rose, rosemary, (sage), (thyme).

Dysmenorrhoea – painful periods:
(Cajeput), calendula, caraway, cardamom, chamomile, clary-sage, (clove), cypress, eucalyptus, fennel, ginger, jasmine, juniper, lavender, lemon, marjoram, melissa, peppermint, pine, rosemary, (sage).

Haemorrhage/menorrhagia – heavy periods:
Chamomile, cypress, eucalyptus, frankincense, geranium, juniper, lemon, myrrh, rose, (sage).

Hypomenorrhoea – scanty periods:
Basil, (hyssop), juniper, lavender, marjoram, melissa, peppermint, rose, rosemary, (sage).

Intramenstrual bleeding – bleeding between periods:
(Cinnamon), cypress, frankincense, geranium, juniper, pine.

Oligomenorrhoea – irregular periods:
Basil, calendula, chamomile, clary-sage, fennel, lavender, melissa, peppermint, rose, (thyme).

Ovarian tonic:
Cypress, (sage).

Premenstrual Syndrome (PMS):
Benzoin, bergamot, cedarwood, chamomile, clary-sage, cypress, fennel, frankincense, geranium, juniper, lavender, melissa, neroli, rose, rosemary, sandalwood.

Sterility:
Bergamot, (cinnamon), clary-sage, (clove), geranium, jasmine, juniper, melissa, neroli, peppermint, rose, (sage).

Thrush – a fungal infection:
Cedarwood, clary-sage, garlic, geranium, lavender, lemon, myrrh, (sage), tea-tree.

Urinary tract infections:
Bergamot, black pepper, (cajeput), chamomile, cedarwood, eucalyptus, fennel, garlic, geranium, juniper, myrtle, niaouli, pine, (sage), sandalwood, tea-tree, (thyme).

Uterine cancer:
Bergamot, eucalyptus, geranium.

Uterine inflammation:
(Hyssop), juniper, lavender, rosemary, (sage), (thyme).

Uterine tonic:
Clary-sage, frankincense, jasmine, melissa, myrrh, rose.

Vaginal irritation:
Bergamot, chamomile, peppermint, (thyme).

Vaginitis – vaginal inflammation:
Chamomile, (thyme).

GLANDULAR CONDITIONS

Adrenal cortex stimulant – stimulates production of corticosteroids:
Basil, geranium, pine, rosemary, (sage).

Balances female sex hormones:
Cypress, sandalwood.
NB Fennel is oestrogenic in action.

Balances hormones in general:
Geranium.

Balance thyroid:
Garlic.

Breast cancer:
Bergamot.

Breast milk – to decrease flow:
Cypress, peppermint, (sage).
– to increase flow:
Caraway, fennel, *jasmine*, lemongrass.

Cracked nipples:
Calendula.

Diabetes (mellitus):
Eucalyptus, *geranium*, juniper, lemon, rosemary.

Glandular fever – infectious viral disease affecting the lymph nodes:
Tea-tree.

Mastitis – sore, heavy breasts:
Geranium, peppermint.

Prostatitis – inflammation of the prostate:
Jasmine, pine.

CONDITIONS RELATED TO THE HEAD

Alopecia – hair loss:
Cedarwood, lavender, melissa, *rosemary*, (sage), (thyme),
ylang-ylang.

Conjunctivitis/blepharitis – inflammation of the conjunctiva/eyelids of the eye:
Chamomile, clary-sage, geranium, *lavender*, lemon, rose.

Dandruff:
Bergamot, *chamomile*, *cedarwood*, geranium, juniper,
lavender, lemon, patchouli, *rosemary*, sandalwood.

Deafness:
Garlic, niaouli, *rosemary.*

Dizziness:
Caraway, *chamomile,* fennel, *lavender,* melissa, peppermint, rosemary, (sage), (thyme).

Earache/otitis – inflammation of the ear:
Basil, (cajeput), *chamomile,* (clove), garlic, (hyssop), *lavender,* lemon, niaouli, *peppermint,* rose, *rosemary.*

Eyesight – weak:
Fennel, *rosemary.*

Fainting:
Basil, black pepper, *chamomile,* (cinnamon), *lavender,* melissa, neroli, *peppermint, rosemary.*

Gingivitis – inflammation of the gums:
Chamomile, cypress, fennel, mandarin, *myrrh,* orange, (sage), tea-tree, (thyme).

Glossitis – inflammation of the tongue:
Bergamot, geranium, *lemon,* (sage).

Gum strengthener:
(Clove), *lavender, lemon,* (sage), (thyme).

Halitosis – bad breath:
Bergamot, cardamom, *lavender,* melissa, *myrrh,* peppermint, rosemary, (thyme).

Headache:
Basil, black pepper, cardamom, *chamomile,* eucalyptus, lavender, *lemon,* (lemongrass), marjoram, melissa, *peppermint,* rose, *rosemary,* rosewood, (sage), (thyme).

Laryngitis – inflammation of the larynx and vocal cords:
Benzoin, (cajeput), *cedarwood,* cypress, eucalyptus, frankincense, geranium, jasmine, *lavender, lemon,* myrrh, niaouli, (sage), sandalwood, (*thyme*).

Loss of sense of smell:
Basil, rosemary.

Loss of voice:
Cypress, lavender, myrrh, rosemary.

Migraine:
Basil, chamomile, eucalyptus, *lavender*, *lemon*, (lemongrass), marjoram, melissa, *peppermint*, pine, *rose*, *rosemary*.

Mumps – a viral infection:
Chamomile, lemon, (thyme).

Nasal polyps – a benign growth in the nose:
Basil.

Nosebleed:
Cypress, frankincense, *lavender*, *lemon*, pine.

Oral thrush/ulcers:
Chamomile, cypress, geranium, *lavender*, *lemon*, myrrh, orange, *rosemary*, (sage), tea-tree, (thyme).

Quinsy – an abscess near the tonsils:
Black pepper, ginger, (hyssop), *lemon*, (thyme).

Rhinitis – inflammation of the lining of the nose:
Basil, eucalyptus, *lavender*, niaouli, (thyme).

Seborrhoea of the scalp – excess oil production by sebaceous glands:
Bergamot, cedarwood, juniper, patchouli.

Sinusitis – inflammation of the sinuses:
Basil, (cinnamon), (clove), eucalyptus, garlic, *lavender*, *lemon*, niaouli, *peppermint*, pine, *rosemary*, tea-tree, (thyme).

Sore throat:
Benzoin, bergamot, (cajeput), *cedarwood*, clary-sage, eucalyptus, geranium, ginger, (hyssop), *lavender*, *lemon*, myrrh, niaouli, *peppermint*, pine, *rosemary*, (sage), sandalwood, tea-tree, (thyme).

Stomatitis – inflammation of the lining of the mouth:
Bergamot, geranium, *lemon*, myrrh, (sage), tea-tree.

Teething:
Chamomile, lavender.

Tonsillitis – inflammation of the tonsils:
Bergamot, garlic, geranium, *lavender*, *lemon*, rosemary, (sage), tea-tree, (thyme).

Tooth abscess:
Chamomile.

Toothache:
Black pepper, (cajeput), (camphor), *chamomile*, (cinnamon), (clove), garlic, juniper, *lemon, peppermint*, (sage), (thyme).

Vertigo:
Basil, black pepper, caraway, *chamomile*, clary-sage, (clove), melissa, *peppermint, rosemary*.

MUSCULAR CONDITIONS

Aching:
Bergamot, *black pepper*, (cajeput), (camphor), caraway, *chamomile*, (clove), *coriander*, eucalyptus, geranium, *ginger, juniper, lavender*, lemon, *marjoram, pine, rosemary*, (sage), (thyme).

Antispasmodic – relieves smooth muscle spasm:
Basil, bergamot, black pepper, (cajeput), (camphor), caraway, cardamom, *chamomile*, (cinnamon), clary-sage, (clove), coriander, cypress, *eucalyptus*, fennel, (hyssop), jasmine, *juniper, lavender, marjoram*, melissa, neroli, orange, peppermint, rose, *rosemary*, (sage), sandalwood, (thyme).

Arthritis/gout:
Basil, *benzoin*, (cajeput), *calendula*, (camphor), caraway, cedarwood, *chamomile*, (clove), *coriander*, cypress, fennel, garlic, *ginger, juniper, lavender*, lemon, *marjoram*, peppermint, *pine, rosemary*, (sage), (thyme).

Cramp:
Basil, *chamomile*, cypress, garlic, mandarin, *marjoram*.

Lack of tone:
Black pepper, cypress, *juniper, lavender*, lemongrass, *rosemary*.

Lumbago – low backache:
Chamomile, geranium (and analgesic oils).

Rheumatism/fibrositis – pain in the muscles or joints/inflammation of back muscles:
Benzoin, *black pepper*, (cajeput), *calendula*, (camphor), caraway, *chamomile*, (cinnamon), (clove), *coriander*, cypress, eucalyptus, garlic, *ginger*, (hyssop), *juniper, lavender*, lemon, *marjoram*, melissa, *pine, rosemary*, (sage), (thyme).

Rheumatoid arthritis:
Benzoin, (cajeput), (camphor), caraway, *chamomile*, (clove), coriander, cypress, *eucalyptus*, garlic, ginger, (hyssop), *juniper*, *lavender*, lemon, *marjoram*, *pine*, *rosemary*, (sage), (thyme).

Rickets – a disease due to vitamin D deficiency:
Pine, *rosemary*, (thyme).

Sprains/strains – injury to a ligament/muscle or tendon:
Calendula, (camphor), *chamomile*, *eucalyptus*, (hyssop), *lavender*, *marjoram*, *rosemary*, (sage), (thyme).

Stiffness:
Marjoram, *rosemary*, (thyme).

Wasting of muscles:
Myrrh.

NEUROLOGICAL CONDITIONS

Convulsions:
Chamomile, clary-sage, *lavender*.

Epilepsy:
Basil, juniper, *lavender*, *rosemary*.

Nerve stimulant:
Eucalyptus, melissa, patchouli, *rosemary*.

Nerve tonic:
Basil, *chamomile*, clary-sage, frankincense, (hyssop), juniper, *lavender*, marjoram, melissa, peppermint, petitgrain, *rosemary*, (sage), (thyme), ylang-ylang.

Neuralgia – severe pain in a nerve:
Basil, *chamomile*, clary-sage, (clove), coriander, eucalyptus, geranium, (hyssop), *lavender*, marjoram, melissa, peppermint, pine, *rosemary*.

Paralysis:
Basil, juniper, *lavender*, peppermint, *rosemary*, (sage).

Sciatica – pain down thigh from lower back:
Cardamom, *chamomile*, *lavender*, melissa, pine.

Tic – involuntary muscle twitch:
Marjoram (and other antispasmodic oils).

RESPIRATORY CONDITIONS

Asthma – breathing difficulties through bronchospasm:
Basil, benzoin, (cajeput), (camphor), clary-sage, (clove),
cypress, eucalyptus, frankincense, garlic, (hyssop), jasmine,
lavender, lemon, marjoram, melissa, myrrh, peppermint, pine,
rosemary, (sage), sandalwood, (thyme).

Breathing – deep and rapid:
Ylang-ylang.

Breathing – shortness of breath:
(Camphor), frankincense, hyssop.

Bronchitis – inflammation of the bronchi:
Basil, benzoin, bergamot, (cajeput), (camphor), cardamom,
cedarwood, (clove), eucalyptus, frankincense, garlic, (hyssop),
lavender, lemon, marjoram, melissa, niaouli, orange,
peppermint, pine, rosemary, (sage), sandalwood, tea-tree,
(thyme).

Bronchitis – chronic:
(Cajeput), eucalyptus, fennel, frankincense, garlic, ginger,
(hyssop), lavender, lemon, myrrh, myrtle, niaouli, peppermint,
pine, rosemary, (sage), sandalwood.

Catarrh:
Basil, benzoin, bergamot, black pepper, cardamom,
cedarwood, chamomile, eucalyptus, fennel, frankincense,
garlic, ginger, (hyssop), jasmine, juniper, lavender, lemon,
marjoram, melissa, myrrh, myrtle, niaouli, peppermint, pine,
rosemary, sandalwood, tea-tree, (thyme).

Colds/chills:
Basil, benzoin, black pepper, (cajeput), (camphor), cedarwood,
(cinnamon), (clove), eucalyptus, garlic, geranium, ginger,
juniper, lavender, lemon, marjoram, melissa, myrrh, niaouli,
orange, peppermint, pine, rosemary, tea-tree, (thyme).

Coughs:
Benzoin, black pepper, (camphor), cardamom, cedarwood,
(cinnamon), cypress, eucalyptus, frankincense, jasmine,
juniper, lavender, lemon, myrrh, niaouli, peppermint,
rosemary, sandalwood, (thyme).

Cough – convulsive:
Clary-sage, cypress, eucalyptus, lavender, pine, (thyme).

Cough – dry and painful:
Benzoin, bergamot, eucalyptus, lavender, sandalwood.

Cough – tickly:
Chamomile, lavender, marjoram, rose.

Diphtheria – contagious bacterial infection affecting the throat:
Bergamot, eucalyptus, garlic, lavender, myrrh, myrtle.

Emphysema:
Basil, cypress, eucalyptus, garlic, (hyssop), jasmine, myrtle, (thyme).

Flu:
Benzoin, black pepper, (camphor), cedarwood, chamomile, (cinnamon), (clove), cypress, eucalyptus, garlic, geranium, juniper, lavender, lemon, niaouli, peppermint, pine, rosemary, (sage), sandalwood, tea-tree, (thyme).

Flu – preventative:
Fennel, frankincense.

Haemoptysis – coughing up blood:
(Cinnamon), cypress, geranium, juniper, pine.

Hayfever:
Chamomile, cypress, eucalyptus, garlic, lavender, lemon, melissa, orange, pine, rose.

Hiccoughs:
Basil, fennel, mandarin, sandalwood.

Pleurisy –inflammation of the pleura around the lungs:
Caraway, (clove), lemon.

Pneumonia – inflammation of the lungs:
(Cajeput), (camphor), eucalyptus, lavender, lemon, niaouli, peppermint, pine, tea-tree.

Tuberculosis – infectious disease caused by a bacillus:
Bergamot, (cajeput), (camphor), eucalyptus, (hyssop), lavender, lemon, myrrh, peppermint, rosemary, sandalwood.

Whooping cough:
Basil, clary-sage, cypress, fennel, (hyssop), lavender, niaouli, rosemary, tea-tree, (thyme).

CONDITIONS RELATED TO THE SKIN

Abscess:
Bergamot, chamomile, garlic, lavender, tea-tree.

Acne:
Bergamot, (cajeput), calendula, (camphor), cedarwood, chamomile, eucalyptus, garlic, geranium, juniper, lavender, lemon, lemongrass, myrtle, neroli, niaouli, patchouli, peppermint, petitgrain, rose, sandalwood, tea-tree.

Animal bites:
Chamomile, fennel, lavender, (sage).

Astringent:
Cedarwood, (cinnamon), clary-sage, cypress, frankincense, geranium, (hyssop), juniper, myrrh, myrtle, patchouli, peppermint, rose, rosemary, (sage), sandalwood.

Athlete's foot/ringworm – contagious fungal infections:
Calendula, garlic, lavender, lemon, myrrh, patchouli, peppermint, tagetes, tea-tree.

Blisters:
Benzoin, lavender, lemon, myrrh.

Boils:
Chamomile, clary-sage, eucalyptus, garlic, juniper, lavender, lemon, myrrh, niaouli, rose, tea-tree, (thyme).

Broken capillaries:
Chamomile, cypress, lavender, lemon, niaouli, peppermint, rose.

Bruises:
Calendula, (camphor), (cinnamon), (clove), fennel, ginger, (hyssop), lavender, marjoram, peppermint, rosemary, (sage).

Bunions – swollen joint at the base of the big toe:
Lavender, marjoram, peppermint.

Burns:
Calendula, chamomile, (camphor), eucalyptus, geranium, lavender, niaouli, patchouli, rosemary, (sage).
(Use lavender for first aid purposes.)

Carbuncle – a collection of boils:
Bergamot, eucalyptus, frankincense, juniper, lavender, rose.

Cellulite:
Black pepper, *cypress, fennel, geranium,* grapefruit, *juniper, lavender, lemon, patchouli, rosemary.*

Chicken pox – an infectious viral disease:
Bergamot, *chamomile, eucalyptus, lavender, tea-tree.*

Chilblains – red itchy swellings usually on fingers or toes:
Benzoin, black pepper, *calendula,* (camphor), *cypress,* garlic, *lavender, lemon,* marjoram.

Corns – hardened skin on or between the toes:
Garlic, *lemon, tea-tree.*

Deodorant:
Benzoin, bergamot, clary-sage, *cypress, eucalyptus, juniper, lavender,* (lemongrass), *neroli, patchouli, petitgrain, pine, rosewood,* (sage), (thyme).

Dermatitis/eczema – inflammation of the skin:
Benzoin, calendula, cedarwood, *chamomile, cypress, geranium,* (hyssop), *jasmine, juniper, lavender, melissa, patchouli, peppermint, rose,* (sage), *sandalwood.*

Eczema – dry:
Geranium, *juniper, lavender.*

Eczema – weeping:
Bergamot, *juniper, myrrh, patchouli.*

Fevers:
Basil, *bergamot,* black pepper, (camphor), *chamomile, cypress, eucalyptus,* garlic, (hyssop), *juniper, lavender, lemon,* (lemongrass), *melissa, patchouli,* peppermint, pine, *rosemary, tea-tree,* (thyme).

Herpes:
Bergamot, *chamomile, eucalyptus, geranium, lavender, lemon, myrrh, patchouli, tea-tree.*

Insect bites and stings:
Basil, (cajeput), (cinnamon), clary-sage, *fennel,* garlic, *lavender, lemon, melissa,* niaouli, (sage), *tea-tree,* (thyme), ylang-ylang.

Insect repellent:
Basil, cedarwood, *cypress, eucalyptus, geranium, lavender, lemon,* (lemongrass), *patchouli,* peppermint.

Lice:
Bergamot, (camphor), (cinnamon), (clove), *eucalyptus,*
geranium, juniper, lavender, lemon, peppermint, pine,
rosemary, tea-tree, (thyme).

Measles/scarlet-fever – an infectious viral disease/bacterial disease:
Bergamot (measles), *chamomile* (measles), (clove), *eucalyptus,*
geranium, (hyssop), *juniper* (measles), *lavender, tea-tree,*
(thyme).

Nails – fungal conditions:
Tagetes.

Obesity:
Bergamot, *fennel,* garlic, grapefruit, *juniper, lemon, patchouli,*
rosemary.

Psoriasis – a red, itchy skin disease:
Bergamot, cedarwood, chamomile, *juniper, lavender,* tagetes.

Regenerative oils:
All essential oils are regenerative, the most powerful however
are:
Calendula, frankincense, garlic, geranium, jasmine, *juniper,*
lavender, lemon, mandarin, *melissa,* myrrh, neroli, *patchouli,*
rose, tea-tree.

(Ringworm – see Athlete's Foot)

Scabies - a parasitic skin infection:
Bergamot, caraway, (cinnamon), (clove), garlic, *lavender,*
lemon, peppermint, *rosemary,* (thyme).

Scars/stretchmarks:
Calendula, chamomile, frankincense, geranium, *juniper,*
lavender, mandarin, myrrh, neroli, *patchouli,* rose, *tea-tree.*

Shingles – a viral infection:
Bergamot, *eucalyptus, geranium, lemon,* peppermint, *tea-tree.*

Skin tonic:
Basil, *chamomile,* (cinnamon), *cypress,* frankincense,
geranium, juniper, lavender, (lemongrass), patchouli, (sage).

Skin types:

Allergic/sensitive:
Chamomile, jasmine, lavender, melissa, neroli, patchouli, rose, sandalwood.

Chapped/cracked:
Benzoin, calendula, chamomile, geranium, lavender, lemon, myrrh, patchouli, rose, sandalwood.

Congested:
Basil, fennel, geranium, lemon, peppermint, rosemary, (sage).

Dry:
Benzoin, chamomile, geranium, jasmine, lavender, neroli, orange, rose, sandalwood, ylang-ylang.

Inflamed – (see also dermatitis/eczema):
Calendula, (camphor), chamomile, clary-sage, frankincense, geranium, lavender, myrrh, patchouli, peppermint, rose, sandalwood, tea-tree.

Irritable:
Benzoin, bergamot, cedarwood, chamomile, jasmine, lavender, melissa, neroli, orange, peppermint, sandalwood.

Mature:
Benzoin, clary sage, cypress, frankincense, lavender, myrrh, neroli, patchouli, rose, sandalwood.

Normal:
Geranium, jasmine, lavender, neroli, rose.

Oily:
Basil, bergamot, (camphor), cedarwood, cypress, fennel, frankincense, geranium, juniper, lavender, lemon, (lemongrass), mandarin, myrtle, neroli, rose, rosemary, sandalwood, ylang-ylang.

Supersensitive:
Chamomile, geranium, jasmine, neroli, rose.

Snakebite:
Basil, (cinnamon), (clove), fennel, juniper, lavender, lemon, tea-tree, (thyme).

Sunburn/sunstroke:
Chamomile, lavender, sandalwood, tea-tree.

Sweating:
Bergamot, clary-sage, (clove), cypress, lemongrass, pine, (sage).

Thread veins:
Calendula, chamomile, cypress, juniper, lemon, rose.

Ulcers/sores:
Bergamot, calendula (ulcers), (camphor), chamomile, clary-sage, (clove), eucalyptus, frankincense, garlic, geranium, juniper, lavender, lemon, myrrh, niaouli, rosemary, (sage), sandalwood, tea-tree, (thyme), ylang-ylang

Verrucae/warts:
Basil, garlic, lemon, tea-tree.

Wounds:
Benzoin, bergamot, (cajeput), calendula, (camphor), chamomile, (clove), eucalyptus, frankincense, garlic, geranium, (hyssop), juniper, lavender, lemon, marjoram, myrrh, niaouli, patchouli, pine, rose, rosemary, (sage), tea-tree, (thyme).

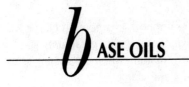

*b*ASE OILS

Basic carrier oils useful in massage are:

corn, grapeseed, olive, peachnut, sesame, soya bean, sunflower, sweet almond.

They must, however, be unrefined, cold pressed and free from additives. Grapeseed is particularly useful as it is colourless, odourless and non-greasy.

Heavier oils can be added to the basic carrier oil in small amounts (up to 10 per cent) to provide extra nourishment to the skin, e.g. apricot kernel, avocado, peach kernel or wheatgerm, or to aid penetration of the essential oils, e.g. avocado and hazelnut.

Wheatgerm is particularly useful as it not only contains vitamin E, but prevents oxidation in oil mixes (by adding 10 per cent to the stock bottle).

Marigold calendula, because of its many therapeutic properties, has been listed for convenience alongside the essential oils. In fact it is a macerated oil and so is added to oil mixes in the same way as the heavier oils (up to 10 per cent).

METHODS OF USING PURE ESSENTIAL OILS

Most essential oils are extracted by steam distillation (citrus oils by expression), whereas those known as 'absolutes' have been extracted by using solvents (including enfleurage). These tend to be more concentrated and may contain impurities from the solvent so should never be taken internally. Gums, or resins, are naturally secreted by the plant. Solvent extraction may be employed to produce resinoids but as neither gums nor resinoids are pure essential oils they should never be taken internally.

Avoid getting the oils near your eyes. If treating the face leave a wide margin around the eyes or apply oils behind the ears instead.

Do not take oils internally without consulting a qualified aromatherapist and never take absolutes, gums or resinoids internally.

Store essential oils and mixes in opaque glass bottles, with an airtight lid, away from direct heat or sunlight and apart from homoeopathic remedies which may be antidoted by the more powerful aromas.

External methods can be used daily for 10 weeks or weekly for 30 weeks after which time a period of 10 days without using oils is recommended.

It is recommended that no more than three or four essential oils should be blended in the same mix.

MASSAGE (carrier oils)

Single application:	Two to three drops of essential oil in a teaspoon (5ml) of carrier oil.
Whole body massage:	Up to eight drops of essential oil in three teaspoons (15ml) of carrier oil.
Stock Bottle:	Fifteen to 30 drops of essential oil in 50ml of carrier oil. Include 5ml of wheatgerm oil to preserve the mix. Including a 'base note' oil can help to fix the aroma.

Children:	Halve the number of drops above. Recommended oils are chamomile, geranium, lavender, mandarin, myrtle, rose, ylang-ylang (or peppermint if diluted down to ¼ or ½ drop).
Babies:	One drop of calendula, chamomile, lavender, mandarin or rose in 50ml of sweet almond oil.

BATHS

Foot or hand bath:	Four to eight drops of essential oils in a bowl of warm water. Soak for 10 minutes and follow if required with localised massage using the same oils.
Full bath:	Five to 10 drops of essential oil in a warm bath. The oils can be dissolved in a teaspoon of bubble bath, vegetable oil or full fat milk. Soak for 10–20 minutes.
Children:	Two to three drops of essential oil dissolved as above.
Babies:	One drop of essential oil dissolved in milk or vegetable oil. (Avoid getting oils in eyes.)

COMPRESS

Put just enough water (hot or cold – see below) into a bowl to be soaked up by the chosen compress (e.g. a flannel). Add four to eight drops of essential oils (half for children). Wring out the compress slightly so that it is wet but not dripping. Place it across the affected area, cover with polythene, then a towel or scarf. Leave for two hours.

Hot water:	Backache, toothache, earache, rheumatic or arthritic pain.

Cold water:	Headache, bruises, sprains, inflammation (hot swellings).

INHALATION

Put six to eight drops of essential oil on a tissue or in a bowl of hot water and inhale for five to 10 minutes keeping your eyes closed. This is not recommended for asthmatics.

Children:	Begin with half the number of drops and only for a few seconds. Increase gradually in subsequent treatments to a maximum of one to two minutes.

INTERNAL MEDICATION

Note: Do not treat children with oils internally.

Medicine:	Put two to three drops of essential oils in a little red wine or honey water (one tsp of honey diluted in one third of a cup of water). Take after food two or three times daily for up to three weeks.
Tea:	Up to three drops of essential oils may be put on one tea bag to make a pot of three to four cups of tea. One cup can be taken up to three times daily (without milk).

MOUTHWASH

Put two to three drops of essential oils in half a cup of warm water or a little brandy/vodka. Stir well before each gargle.

FIRST AID

Burns:	Apply one to two drops of undiluted lavender oil to the burn (once or twice only).
Cuts:	One to two drops of undiluted lemon oil applied to a cut will stop bleeding.
Cold sores:	One drop of undiluted eucalyptus and/or lemon oils may be applied once or twice. Mix oils in lotion/oil in subsequent applications.
Bites and stings:	Apply one drop of undiluted lavender or lemon (diluted in a little water for children).

ROOM FRESHENER

Put six to 10 drops of essential oils in a burner or small bowl of water (put in a warm place).

PETS

Sponge down pets with water containing three to four drops of essential oils for fleas, mange, fevers, etc. It is advisable that guidance is sought from a professional aromatherapist before essential oils are applied to pets.

ALPHABETICAL INDEX OF CONDITIONS

A

Abdominal distension	75
Abscess	90
Acid stomach	75
Acne	90
Adrenal cortex stimulant oils	82
Air swallowing	75
Alcohol poisoning	73
Allergies	71, 93
Alopecia	83
Anaemia	73
Analgesic oils	71
Anaphrodisiac oils	78
Anger	78
Angina	73
Animal bites	90
Anorexia nervosa	78
Anti-cancer oils	71
Anti-inflammatory oils	71
Antiseptic oils	71
Antispasmodic oils	71, 86
Anti-viral oils	71
Anxiety	78
Aphrodisiac oils	78
Appetite – to increase	77
Arteriosclerosis	73
Arthritis	86
Asthma	88
Astringent oils	90
Athlete's foot	90

B

Back pain (lumbago)	86
Balancing oils	71

Bedwetting   79
Bites and stings – insect   91
Blepharitis   83
Blisters   90
Blood cholesterol – high   73
Blood sugar – high   73
Blood purifier oils   73
Body temperature – high   73
Body temperature – low   73
Boils   90
Breast cancer   83
Breast milk – to decrease   83
Breast milk – to increase   83
Breathing – deep and rapid   88
Breathing – shortness of breath   88
Broken capillaries   90
Bronchitis   88
Bronchitis – chronic   88
Bruises   90
Bunions   90
Burns   90

C

Cancer   71
Carbuncles   90
Catarrh   88
Cellulite   91
Chicken pox   91
Chilblains   91
Chills   88
Cholera   75
Circulation – poor   74
Colds   88
Colic   75
Colitis   75
Concentration – poor   80

Confusion	79
Conjunctivitis	83
Constipation	75
Convulsions	87
Cooling oils	72
Corns	91
Cough	88
Cough – convulsive	89
Cough – dry and painful	89
Cough – tickly	89
Cracked nipples	83
Cramp	86
Cystitis	80

D

Dandruff	83
Deafness	84
Deodorant	91
Depression	79
Dermatitis	91
Detoxifying oils	72
Diabetes	83
Diarrhoea	76
Digestive stimulant oils	76
Diphtheria	89
Diuretic oils	80
Dizziness	84
Dysentry	76

E

Earache	84
Eczema	91
Eczema – dry	91
Eczema – weeping	91

Emphysema 89
Epilepsy 87
Exhaustion 79
Eyesight – weak 84

F

Fainting 84
Fear 79
Female sex hormones – to balance 83
Fevers 91
Fibrositis 86
Flatulence 76
Flu 89
Flu – preventative 89
Fluid retention 80
Food poisoning 76
Frigidity 80
Fungicidal oils 72

G

Gallstones 76
Gastralgia 76
Gastritis 76
Gastroenteritis 76
Gingivitis 84
Glandular fever 83
Glossitis 84
Gonorrhoea 80
Gout 86
Grief 79
Gum strengthener oils 84

H

Haemoptysis   89
Haemorrhage   74, 81
Haemorrhoids   77
Haemostatic oils   72
Halitosis   84
Hayfever   89
Headache   84
Heartburn   77
Heart tonic oils   74
Hepatitis   77
Herpes   91
Hiccoughs   89
Hormones – to balance   83
Hypersensitivity   79
Hypertension   74
Hypotension   74
Hysteria   79

I

Immune system stimulant oils   74
Impatience   79
Impotence   80
Incontinence   81
Indecision   79
Indigestion   77
Inflammation   71
Insect repellent   91
Insomnia   79
Intestinal infections   77
Intramenstrual bleeding   82
Irritability   79

J

Jaundice   77
Jealousy   80

K

Kidneys – inflamed   81
Kidneys – stones   81
Kidneys – tonic oils   81

L

Laryngitis   84
Leucorrhoea   81
Lice   92
Liver – cirrhosis   77
Liver – congestion   77
Liver – tonic oils   77
Loss of sense of smell   84
Loss of voice   84
Lymphatic congestion   74
Lymph nodes – swollen or inflamed   74

M

Malaria   74
Mastitis   83
Measles   92
Memory – poor   80
Menopause   81
Menstruation – Amenorrhoea   81
              Dysmenorrhoea   81
              Hypomenorrhoea   81
              Menorrhagia   81

Menstruation – Oligomenorrhoea 82
Migraine 85
Mumps 85
Muscle spasm 86
Muscular aches 86
Muscular wasting 87
Muscular – lack of tone 86
Muscular – stiffness 87

N

Nails – Fungal conditions 92
Nasal polyps 85
Nausea 77
Nerve stimulant oils 87
Nerve tonic oils 87
Neuralgia 87
Nosebleed 85

O

Obesity 92
Oral thrush 85
Otitis 84
Ovarian tonic oils 82

P

Pain relief (see analgesic) oils 71
Palpitations 74
Panic 79
Paralysis 87
Paranoia 79
Pleurisy 89
Pneumonia 89

Premenstrual syndrome 82
Prostatitis 83
Psoriasis 92

Q

Quinsy 85

R

Regenerative oils 92
Relaxing oils 72
Rheumatism 86
Rheumatoid arthritis 87
Rhinitis 85
Rickets 87
Ringworm 90
Run down 80

S

Scabies 92
Scalp – seborrhoea 85
Scarlet fever 92
Scars 92
Sciatica 87
Sedative oils 72
Shingles 92
Shock 80
Sinusitis 85
Skin – allergies/sensitive 93
    chapped/cracked 93
    congested 93
    dry 93

	inflamed	93
	irritable	93
	mature	93
	normal	93
	oily	93
	supersensitive	93
	tonic	92
	ulcers	94
Snakebite		93
Sores		94
Sore throat		85
Spleen tonic oils		74
Sprains		87
Sterility		82
Stimulant oils		72
Stomach tonic oils		77
Stomatitis		85
Strains		87
Stress		78
Stretchmarks		92
Sunburn		94
Sunstroke		94
Sweating		94

T

Teething	85
Thread veins	94
Thrush	82
Thyroid balancing oils	83
Tic	87
Tonic oils	72
Tonsillitis	85
Tooth abscess	85
Toothache	86
Travel sickness	78
	89
	78

U

Ulcers – digestive 78
Ulcers – mouth 85
Ulcers – skin 94
Uplifting oils 73
Urinary tract infections 82
Uterine cancer 82
Uterine inflammation 82
Uterine tonic oils 82

V

Vaginal irritation 82
Vaginitis 82
Varicose veins 74
Vasoconstrictor oils 75
Verrucae 94
Vertigo 86
Viruses 71
Vomiting 78

W

Warming oils 73
Warts 94
White blood cells – to stimulate 75
Whooping cough 89
Worms 78
Wounds 94

*i*NDEX OF ESSENTIAL OILS BY FAMILY AND PRINCIPAL CHEMICAL CONSTITUENTS

Key to suffixes of chemicals:
Terpenes – 'ene
Alcohols – 'ol
Ketones – 'one
Aldehydes – 'yde
Esters   – 'yl, 'ate

Class: CONIFERAE

Family: CUPRESSACEAE (Conifer family)

Cypress	Cedrol, d-pinene, d-camphene, terpinyl esters, cymene, terpenic alcohol
Juniper	Terpineol, alpha-pinene, cadinene, camphene, junene, camphor of juniper

Family: PINACEAE (Conifer family)

Cedarwood	Cedrene, cedrol, cedrenol
Pine (needle)	Bornyl acetate, borneol

Class: MONOCOTYLEDONS

Family: GRAMINEAE (Aromatic grasses)

Lemongrass	Citral (70–80 per cent), myrcene (15–20 per cent)

Family: LILIACEAE (Lily family)

Garlic	Allicin, disulphides

Family: ZINGIBERACEAE (Ginger family)

Cardamom	Terpineol, cineol, limonene
Ginger	Zingiberene, zingiberol, camphene, phellandrene, cineol, borneol, linaloöl, citral

Class: DICOTYLEDONS

Family: ANONACEAE (Magnolia family)

Ylang-ylang	Alcohols and esters (50–60 per cent), sesquiterpenes (35 per cent). See also page 68.

Family: BURSERACEAE (Resinous trees and shrubs)

Frankincense	Pinene, dipentene, p-cymene, camphene, d-borneol, verbenone, verbenol
Myrrh	Pinene, dipentene, limonene, cadinene, eugenol, formic acid, acetic acid, myrrholic acid, aldehydes, alcohols, resins

Family: COMPOSITAE (Daisy family)

Chamomile	Esters (85 per cent), chamazulene
Tagetes (Marigold)	Tagetone (60–70 per cent), other ketones (5–10 per cent), limonene, ocymene

Family: GERANIACEAE (Geranium family)

Geranium	Geraniol, citronellol, linaloöl, terpineol

Family: LABIATAE (Mint family)

Basil	Methyl chavicol (40–50 per cent), linaloöl, cineol, pinene, camphor
Clary-sage	Linaloöl, linalyl acetate
Hyssop	Pinocamphone, pinene
Lavender	Linalyl acetate, linaloöl, geraniol, lavandulol, pinene, cineol, caryophyllene, coumarin
Marjoram	Terpinene, terpineol, terpinen-4-ol, pinene
Melissa	Linaloöl, geraniol, citronellol, citral, citronellal
Patchouli	Patchouli alcohol, terpenes, benzaldehyde, eugenol, cinnamic aldehyde
Peppermint	Menthol (40–60 per cent), limonene, menthone, cadinene, phellandrene, pinene

Rosemary	Cineol, borneol, pinene, camphene, camphor, dipentene, caryophyllene
Sage	Thujone (40–60 per cent), borneol (10–15 per cent), bornyl acetate, salvene, pinene, cineol, camphor
Thyme	Thymol and carvacrol (60 per cent)

Family: LAURACEAE (Laurel family)

Camphor	Camphor, linaloöl, terpineol, pinene, limonene, cineol, safrole, methyl eugenol, caryophyllene, terpenes
Cinnamon	Cinnamic aldehyde, eugenol
Rosewood	Linaloöl (80–90 per cent), terpineol, nerol, geraniol

Family: MYRTACEAE (Shrubs and trees)

Cajeput	Cineol (45–65 per cent), terpineol, pinene, aldehydes
Clove	Eugenol (70–90 per cent), eugenol acetate, caryophyllene
Eucalyptus	Cineol (70–80 per cent), eucalyptol, pinene, aldehydes, terpenes, globulol
Myrtle	Myrtenol, cineol, pinene, geraniol
Niaouli	Cineol (50–60 per cent), terpineol, pinene, benzaldehyde
Tea-tree	Pinene, cymene, cineol, terpenes, terpinene, alcohols

Family: OLEACEAE (Olive family)

Jasmine	Benzyl acetate (65 per cent), linaloöl, linalyl acetate, benzyl alcohol, jasmone, indole, methyl anthranilate

Family: PIPERACEAE (Pepper family)

Black pepper   Piperine

Family: ROSACEAE (Rose family)

Rose   Phenylethyl alcohol (60–70 per cent), citronellol (20 per cent), geraniol and nerol (13 per cent)

Family: RUTACEAE (Citrus family)

Bergamot   Linalyl acetate, limonene, linaloöl
Grapefruit   Limonene, citral
Lemon   Terpenes (95 per cent), limonene, camphene, pinene, geraniol, citral, linaloöl
Mandarin   Limonene, methyl anthranilic acid, methyl ester
Neroli   Linalyl acetate (7 per cent), linaloöl (30 per cent), terpineol, nerol, geraniol and acetates (10 per cent), pinene
Orange   d-limonene (90 per cent), linalyl acetate, linaloöl, terpineol, citral
Petitgrain   Linaloöl (40 per cent), linalyl acetate (50 per cent)

Family: SANTALACEAE (Sandalwood family)

Sandalwood   Santalol (90 per cent), santalene, santalone, santene, santenone, santenol, acids and aldehydes

Family: UMBELLIFERAE (Parsley family)

Caraway   Carvone (50–60 per cent), limonene
Coriander   Coriandrol (d-linaloöl) (60–65 per cent), pinene, terpinene, cymene, borneol, geraniol
Fennel   Anethole (50–70 per cent), d-phellandrene, d-limonene

𝓤 SEFUL ADDRESSES

For mail order supplies of aromatherapy products, or to book yourself onto a training course, contact:

Shirley Price Aromatherapy Ltd
Essentia House
Upper Bond Street
Hinckley
Leics LE10 1RS
United Kingdom

General enquiries Tel: 01455-615466
Product orders Tel: 01455-615436
Training courses Tel: 01455-633231
Fax: 01455-615054

For lists of accredited practitioners, to become a member of a professional body yourself, or to enquire about standards required for the accreditation of courses, contact:

The International Society of Professional Aromatherapists (ISPA)
ISPA House
82 Ashby Road
Hinckley
Leics LE10 1SN
United Kingdom
Tel: 01455-637987
Fax: 01455-890956